FRUMPY 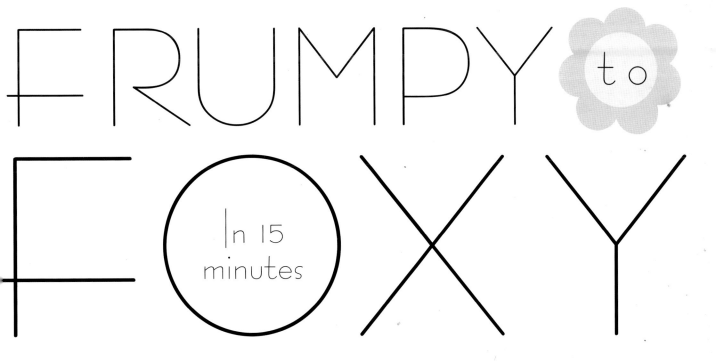 to

FOXY

In 15 minutes

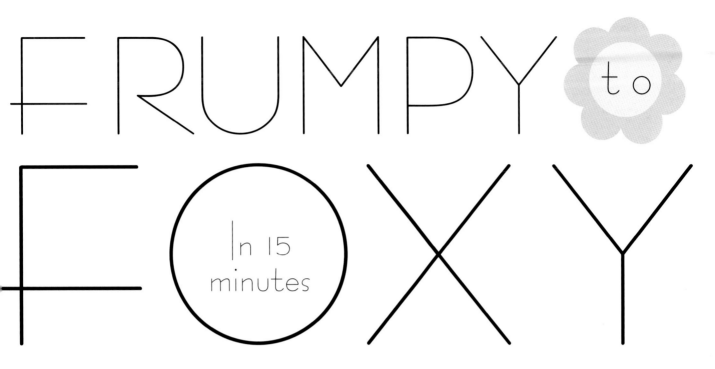

FRUMPY to FOXY

In 15 minutes

style tips for every woman

ELYCIA RUBIN & RITA MAUCERI

APPLE

TEXT © 2005 BY ELYCIA RUBIN AND RITA MAUCERI

PUBLISHED IN THE UK IN 2005 BY
APPLE PRESS
SHERIDAN HOUSE
112-116A WESTERN ROAD
HOVE
EAST SUSSEX BN3 1DD
ENGLAND
WWW.APPLE-PRESS.COM

10 9 8 7 6 5 4 3 2 1

ISBN 1-84543-017-4

COVER AND BOOK DESIGN BY LAURA MCFADDEN
ILLUSTRATIONS BY BARBARA MCGREGO4R/WWW.ARTSCOUNSELINC.COM

PRINTED AND BOUND IN SINGAPORE

Dedication

We dedicate this book to our mothers, Andrea & Gladys, and to Gram Bev & Tray – the four foxiest ladies around. We'd be forever frumpy without your love and inspiration. xoxo

Contents

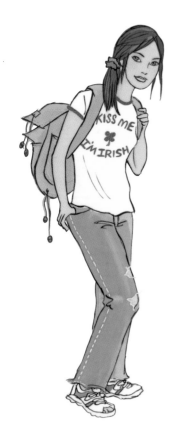

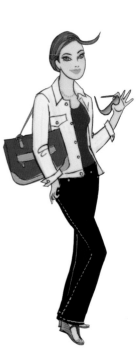

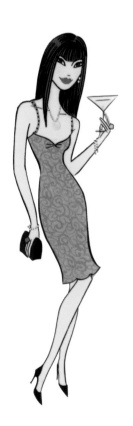

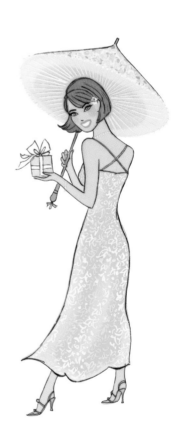

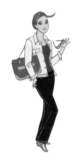 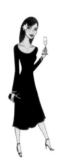 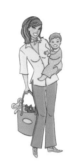 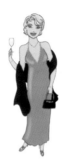 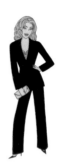 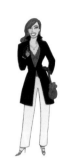

Acknowledgments

~ Thanks to the foxy ladies at Fair Winds Press: Holly Schmidt, Rhiannon Soucy, Brigid Carroll, Mary Aarons, Janelle Randazza, and Claire MacMaster—and at Lifetime Media: Karen Kelly, Cathy Repetti, and Jacqueline Varoli Grace.

~ Prince Steven Cojocaru (one of the foxiest guys on the planet)—we love and adore you to pieces!

~ Paula Munier, Dalyn Miller, and Adam Nelson, thank you for your support and guidance.

~ Barbara McGregor, thank you for bringing the foxy girl to life.

~ Audie England, thank you for your foxy photographs.

~ Christy Fowler, thank you for your irresistible creativity.

~ Heidi Weisel, your foxy designs inspire us season after season.

~ Andrew Steinberg and Gina Rugolo Judd, thank you for your encouragement.

~ Xs and Os to our biggest fans, Brad Kaplan and Mark Mauceri—even when we're at our frumpiest, you still think we're foxy.

~ To our family and friends, thank you for your love: Jim Kofalt, Norm Rubin, Rosalyn Rubin, Jeff Rubin, Alan Sitomer, Shane Rubin, Jarrett Rubin, Molly Craig, Julia Cobb.

~ To our talented friends, thank you for your support: Jeanine Lobell, Carineh Martin, Lis Röhm, Ole Henriksen, Bobbi Brown, Melissa Garfola, Frederic Fekkai, Cara Maiman, Jennifer Mayer, Alison Brod, Monique Lhuillier, Susan Ashbrook, Renata Espinosa, Celine Kaplan, Sally Horchow, Suze Yalof Schwartz, Jason Newman, and Carmen Electra.

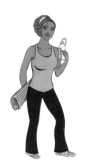 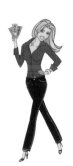 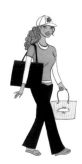 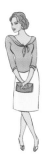 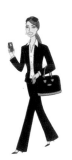 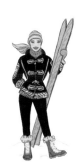

Foreword

If there was ever a true "frump collides with fox" story, it's mine and Elycia's. Take one frizzy-haired Hollywood newcomer obsessed with fashion (that would be moi) and one devastatingly poised fox (Miss. Elycia, naturally), and somehow an unlikely yet beautiful friendship was born.

But forget Elycia being my muse; over the years we have trafficked in enough secret, whispered beauty exchanges to make heads spin. That's why it came as no surprise to hear that Elycia and Rita were cooking up this très cool style bible. With their innate charm and accessibility, I couldn't think of a better duo to share their expertise than these two fast lane foxettes.

Of course it's not a bad idea for me to swap trade secrets with them since Elycia and Rita have a few tricks up their sleeves when it comes to pulling it together … without falling apart. Want to know how to cut forty frantic minutes of getting ready into a manageable fifteen? Stumped on what to pack to look tantalizing on a tropical getaway? Wondering if that micro mini might be a tragic faux pas at the office? Need to know how to tame a wild mane or avoid a time-sucking face full of makeup? These girls really let it spill, spill, spill. Their revealing style secrets will transform even the most disheveled damsel into one divine dish.

So I do hope you take to heart the wise and wonderful musings of these Girl Scouts of glamour. Because sprucing up the planet one outfit at a time is truly a foxy thing to do.

—STEVEN COJOCARU, STYLE EXPERT, *THE TODAY SHOW* CONTRIBUTOR, *ENTERTAINMENT TONIGHT* AND *THE INSIDER* CORRESPONDENT, AND AUTHOR OF *RED CARPET DIARIES: CONFESSIONS OF A GLAMOUR BOY*

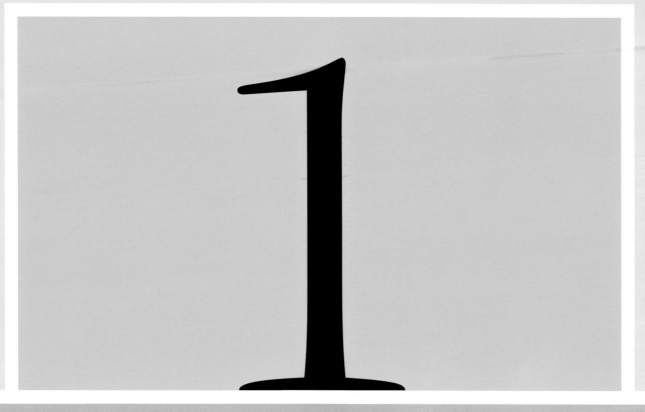

1

Foxy Beginnings

Get Foxified

~Get Foxified~

These days, life often feels like one big scramble. You force yourself out of bed, gulp down a double latte, rush to work, dash to after-work activities, and cram weekends full of workouts, errands, movies, dinner dates, family outings, and endless other things. It's a struggle to keep yourself looking half-way pulled together, much less foxy. And sometimes it's just easier to succumb to the frumps—those inevitable frizzy hair days, blotchy skin days, big and bloated days, or schlumpy sweats and slippers days. Everyone gets them!

Getting dressed should be fun, but day after day it starts to feel like a chore and a bit of a bore. You know the drill . . . standing at your closet with a blank expression on your face and without a clue what to wear. Ring a bell? You want to look foxy, but you don't have the time to put it together. At times it's easier to just give up.

That's when you fall into the frumps.

Some days we wish there were a phone booth we could just dash into, count to ten, and come out totally transformed, but, alas, that only happens in the movies. In real life, there are no phone booths, no fairy godmothers, and no twenty-four hour swat teams of Hollywood specialists to help us look our best.

Our inspiration for writing this book was our own manic lives. In our quest to be forever foxy, we searched high and low for answers to that all-important question: How can we be stylish in a snap without spending a starlet's ransom? After years of spending hours in the bathroom nearly every day with the curling iron in one hand and a gallon of mousse in the other, waiting for our nails to dry and our greasy body lotion to finally sink in, we discovered tricks that make getting ready as simple as possible. After much fine-tuning, we came up with a Foxy Formula.

The result is *Frumpy to Foxy in 15 Minutes Flat,* a handbook to suit every occasion of your daily life.

In life, there may be times when you don't have the drive to get foxified, or when you wonder what's the point when you're just hanging at home. But if it were really easy, who wouldn't want to look foxy all the time? How could you resist! Whether you're dining out or lounging in, do it with a foxy spin, and bid a final fond farewell to the frumps.

Being foxy may sound like something it takes years, beaucoup bucks, or a jackpot gene pool to achieve. But the truth is that regardless of your shapely size, or the size of your pocketbook, all it takes is a few proven tricks to bring out your inner fox. If you think foxy is those va-va-voom girls you see in men's magazines, think again. You are foxy, and even if you don't look it now, we'll show you how to bring out that inner style.

The sweet little secret? Becoming foxy doesn't have to take a lot of time, effort, or money. If you know

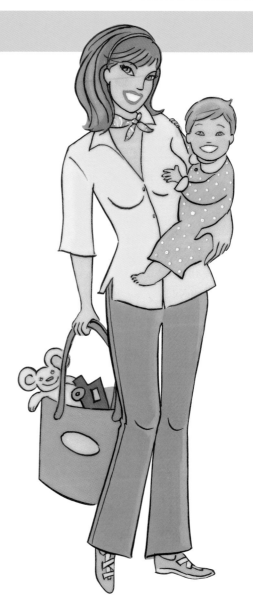

the right shortcuts, it takes just fifteen minutes a day. Trust us, we've done the "clinical trials" and we're thrilled to report it's doable. If you're not a believer, then read on, Foxy, and you can thank us later!

Building a Foxy Base

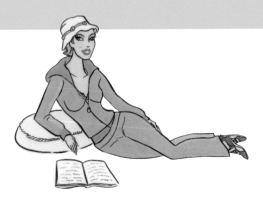

From work to weekends to Sunday sweats, all it takes is fifteen minutes to go from frumpy to foxy. The trick is building the right base: It'll save you tons of time and make the difference between fifteen minutes and fifty. And you aren't the only one who'll benefit—your friends and family will thank us. Now when you yell out "I'll be ready in two minutes!" it'll really be just thirteen more, instead of thirty.

First, a few ground rules. The foxy formula takes just fifteen minutes *if* you have a good base to start with—otherwise, we can't be held responsible! To break it down, that leaves five minutes to dress, five minutes for hair, and five minutes to put on your foxy face.

Some special occasions may lend themselves to a little Foxy Overtime if you can spare it—weddings, black-tie galas, or any affair where you want to get more dolled up than usual. But for most occasions in your day-to-day life, it shouldn't take more than fifteen minutes to foxify and go.

The one thing not included in those fifteen minutes is shower time, since that's variable. For all we know, you could be the type of gal who likes to sing the entire first act of *Hairspray* while showering.

Here are all the essentials you'll need to create a solid base. Some should be done on a weekly basis, others monthly or occasionally, but if you make them a regular habit, they'll become the building blocks for everyday foxiness.

~Foxy Face~

There's no use slapping makeup onto your mug if it's not clean and fresh to begin with. Exposed to sun, wind, pollution, and partying, your foxy face has enough of an uphill battle, so give yourself an edge with the right skin-care basics.
• Every time you wash your face, use a washcloth for a more thorough cleansing, especially at night when you want to get rid of the day's grime. Follow a warm water wash with a splash of cold to tighten pores. Use a gentle cleanser like Cetaphil or Neutrogena Extra Gentle, affordable drugstore brands that have earned raves from foxettes everywhere.
• Every day, use a moisturizer with an SPF of 30 or higher, and don't forget to cover your neck and chest. Oil of Olay's daytime creams with sunscreen smell fresh and sink right in.

Foxy Time-Saver If you use a tinted moisturizer with SPF, you can condense three steps (moisturizer, sunscreen, foundation) into one.

• Once a week, use a gentle exfoliator to peel away those frumpy flakes. Look for a super-fine gentle scrub; the ones with thick chunks of crushed almonds or apricot seeds don't quite cut it—and could end up cutting you.

• Once a month, give yourself an at-home facial with a quickie steam and mask. To open up pores, cover your face for a few minutes with a washcloth that has been soaked in warm water. Follow with a mask—clay for oily skin and clogged pores, or sea-weed for moisturizing.

Foxy Time-Saver Don't have time to run to the drugstore and get a mask? Try one of these quick and easy at-home concoctions: dry oatmeal mixed with honey and egg yolk to exfoliate; olive oil mixed with raw egg and honey to nourish; avocado with olive oil and a few drops of chamomile oil to moisturize.

• To keep your skin plumped and dewy year-round, and to combat all those evil elements that are tough on skin, get a humidifier. We love having one in the bedroom, and a mini one in the office.

• Fill a small spray container with bottled water and fresh mint leaves, or spike the water with a dash of witch hazel and geranium oil. Keep it in the fridge for moments when your skin needs a boost. Spritz all over to wake up your skin—and your senses.

~Shower Savvy~

Usually your eyes are still half closed as you stumble into the shower. But with a little foxy know-how, you can make the most of that daily rinse and ensure that your precious time doesn't go down the drain.

• Use warm water rather than hot. A steaming soak may feel good but can dry out your skin.

Foxy Time-Saver While your skin is nice and moist in the shower, gently push back your cuticles for cleaner-looking nails.

• Once a week, exfoliate using a gentle body scrub while you're rinsing off. Doing this in the shower rather than the tub will save you time and mess.

Foxy Tip For a smooth neckline, combine one part brown sugar with one part body gel and mas-sage mixture onto wet chest and shoulders. Rinse.

~Moisture Mania~

Keep that foxy bod lubed up, and you'll be glowing. You should keep two body moisturizers on hand: one for day and one for evening.

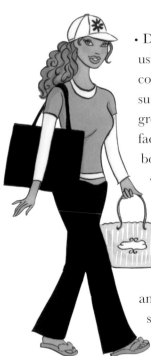

• During the day, save time by using a body lotion that's a combination moisturizer and sunscreen. (Lubriderm makes a great version.) You protect your face from the sun, so treat your body with the same TLC.

• At night, you want something heavier to replenish your skin while you sleep. Anything with shea butter is a good bet. L'Occitane's version is unbelievably rich and creamy and will make your skin feel the same. Foxettes also love to raid their local drugstores for Palmer's Cocoa Butter Formula, which does wonders for dry heels and elbows.

• After showering, pat your skin with a towel, leaving it still damp. Douse moisturizer all over your body to capture that dewiness. Moisturizing within the first few minutes after you step out of the shower or bath is key because it traps those precious beads of H_2O. Plus, it gives your lotion a few minutes to sink in while you indulge in the rest of your speedy morning or evening routine.

Foxy Time-Saver: Skip perfume and use a hydrating body lotion that includes a light fragrance. Nivea has a clean, irresistible scent. For a little extra money, Laura Mercier and Jo Malone also make delicious lotions that last and last.

• Foxettes love fast-absorbing body oils that reflect light and soften imperfections. Dry body oils come in spray form, which saves time. Just rub them in with a quick swipe, and you'll have none of the leftover greasiness that comes with heavier lotions.

Our all-time faves are L'Occitane Protective Body Oil and Neutrogena Sesame Oil. They sink right in and smell heavenly.

~Tan-O-Matic~

We like the tanned look because it evens out skin tone and camouflages any flaws. Self-tanners are super affordable and easy to use, and they give you that just-back-from-the-beach glow without the leathery UV damage. Neutrogena and L'Oréal make natural-looking tanners; for extra indulgence, try Clarins or Lancôme. When you want to really go for the gold, opt for spray-on tans at salons which last about a week.

~Do Deodorize~

No explanation needed here. Foxy girls have to smell sweet. Choose a clear roll-on or solid that won't leave frumpy white smears on your clothing.

~Razor's Edge~

Shave every other day, or as needed. It's a minor hassle, but it takes two minutes and has major foxy payoffs. Shave at night while you're taking a bath—it's easier and saves you from feeling harried (and hairy) in the morning. On those occasions when you wake and realize that you forgot to shave, don't resort to dry shaving. You could end up with a mess of irritating bumps. Instead, lubricate your legs with body oil, then shave while occasionally dipping the razor in water to clean it. When you're done, just rub in the leftover oil. Stubbly to silky in seconds!

Foxy Tip: The next time you're standing in the shower allowing your conditioner to sit on your hair for a few minutes before you rinse, use some of it to shave your legs at the same time.

~Wax Away~

There's no delicate way to deal with the topic of bikini hair. And let's be honest, less is more. Whether you fancy bikini or Brazilian, wax every six weeks or shave as often as needed. Keep an eye on your upper lip, too, and don't let that pesky fuzz creep up.

Foxy Tip: If you are traveling and suddenly realize you're overdue for a wax, do-it-yourself waxing strips can work in a pinch until you can make it to the salon. Or in an emergency, just pluck those pesky strays with a tweezer.

~Bleach Baby~

Too much dark hair in the wrong places can look a little grizzly, and while waxing or shaving is an option, bleaching is easy and lasts a good while. If you're bleaching an area on your face, make sure you use a gentle formula.

Foxy Tip: Don't bleach those brows. They could end up platinum, when what you wanted was golden brown. Have the pro who shapes your brows or colors your hair do it. He or she will know how to get just the right shade.

~Nifty Nails ~

Neat-looking nails are a must for foxy girls, so try to get a professional manicure once a month. In between, use these tips to keep your fingertips looking fab.
• Don't let nails get too long. They are much more likely to break or look beat-up. Keep about one-eighth inch of white tip showing, and file each nail into a rounded-edge square shape.
• When you don't have time to get to the salon, try this Foxy Five-Minute Manicure. File nails. Soak fingers for 30 seconds in a bowl of warm water spiked with lavender oil. Push back cuticles and clean under nails using a wooden orange stick. Rub hand lotion onto cuticles to neaten them up. Rub each nail bed with a slice of fresh lemon to clean off residue and help bleach out any spots. Finish off with a coat of quick-drying clear polish like Nailtiques.
• Keep a can of quick-dry nail spray or nail-drying oil on hand. It's pure genius when you're in a hurry.

Foxy Time-Saver: For an alternative to polish, buff your nails to a sexy shine using a dab of buffing cream and a buffing file.

~Banish Bumps~

Blemishes are a frumpy fact of life. Whenever you feel a little bugger creeping up, have a bottle of Industrial-strength zapper on hand, like Oxy Cream or Epicuren Lancer Gel.

Foxy Tip: In an emergency before going out, try holding an ice cube on that red puffer to reduce swelling, then pat on some rubbing alcohol. Overnight, dab on some mint toothpaste to help dry it up.

~Twinkle Toes~

We're not embarrassed to say that we have a secret fetish for foxy feet. Put your best foot forward by keeping them pretty and polished to flatter those sexy sandals and playful peep toes.

• Once a month, indulge in a salon pedicure, or give yourself one at home. Soak feet for five minutes in a big bowl of warm water with peppermint oil. Exfoliate with a store-bought foot scrub, or make your own using olive oil and sea salt. Blend and rub all over your tootsies, especially on heels and toes. Pat your feet dry and polish—base coat, two thin layers of color, and a clear top coat. Foxy feet in no time!

• To make life easy, keep polish feminine but subtle. During warmer months, a pale pink or sheer beige looks foxy on all skin tones and goes with anything. When it gets cooler, try a deep burgundy color. A French pedicure also holds up well and goes with everything, and unlike dark polish, you won't notice every little chip.

Foxy Tip: Use a foot cream with alpha hydroxy acids to get rid of scaly skin.

~Pearly Whites~

Our favorite foxy accessory is a great smile, so always start the day (and end it) with a thorough minty flossing and brushing. Every couple of months, try a whitening treatment from your local drugstore. And be sure to keep mints or peppermint drops on hand at all times. The frumpiest of frumps is blasting someone with foul breath.

~Brow Beat~

The right pair of eyebrows can make a foxy face. Whether you pluck them yourself or get them done at a salon, keep them shaped. Foxy girls have thick, solid brows with a defined arch. Before you let a professional have her way with your brows, do a little research. Talk to friends and get personal recommendations. If the stylist over-plucks, you could wind up with brow bald spots. Once you get a foxy shape, it's easy for you to maintain it at home.

~Eye-C-U~

We all rise with puffy eyes from time to time. When you do, give them a little intensive care. To help wake them up, keep a warm washcloth lightly pressed over your eyes, then follow with a cold compress for a few minutes. Dab on a refreshing gel, such as Origins No Puffery. Dry, itchy eyes are also frumpy, so keep some moisturizing drops around.

~Cosmetics Counter~

You can buy almost everything you need to foxify yourself at the drugstore. You don't need to spend $150 on a jar of beauty cream! Lower-priced brands are super savvy these days and offer many of the same cutting-edge ingredients as the fancier ones. Still, filling your makeup bag with all the essentials can add up quickly if you splurge on the wrong things, so here are a few guidelines to keep you foxy and flush.

• Whenever it's comfortable for you, indulge on foundations, facial serums, and exfoliators. Pricier foundations tend to offer better blending, consistency, and a wider range of shades. Quality facial serums have advanced technology behind them and more sophisticated ingredients. And we haven't found a low-priced exfoliator yet that's quite as gentle and refined as the more costly ones. Facial skin is one area foxettes don't want to mess with.

• To get extra bang for your buck, look for products that are two-in-one: two-sided lip pencils; toothpaste as blemish cream; body lotion to tame frizzies; bug spray with SPF; Vaseline to mold brows and soften feet, elbows, and lips; baby oil to moisturize legs, soften cuticles, tame split ends, and remove eye makeup.

~Making Up~

It's never a great idea to put on your face as you're behind the wheel, driving thirty miles per hour. So we've boiled the tedious task of makeup down to a super quick five-minute routine that will give you a basic, fabulous face. We call it *the Foxy Five:* **cover-up, powder, blush, mascara, and lipstick.**

• Start with a sheer to medium cover-up with sunscreen built in. We prefer sticks or compacts because we can apply them quickly and easily. Follow with a few extra swipes under your eyes, around your nose, and anywhere else you have blotches. Dust on a light translucent powder—oil-free if you tend to shine. Next is blush: neutral pink for fair skin, peach for medium skin, or bronze for olive skin. Finish off with a quick coat of mascara, and your favorite shade of lip gloss for the perfect pout.

• Lipsticks, tinted lip balms, and glosses are must-haves for any foxy face—how can a girl laugh and pout without? But you don't need fifty different lipsticks. Choose three shades that you like: one for work, one for evenings out, and one for special occasions. Try a pinky nude for everyday, a berry or dusty rose for going out, and a wine or sultry red for more lavish affairs.

Foxy Tip: Create your own shade. Coat your lips with a colorless balm, dab on neutral liner, and blend with your finger.

• Eyes should always be a foxy focal point. Accentuate them by sweeping white or silver shimmer on the lids, or lining the inside corners with soft white pencil to open them up.

Foxy Tip: Because they give an instant "eye lift," we love lash curlers. Afterward, apply brown or black mascara close to the roots, then bat away!

• Take advantage of those brilliant multi-purpose all-in-one makeup sticks that work on lips, eyes, and cheeks. Choose a neutral color like bronze, rose, or peach. Talk about a foxy time-saver!

~Lovely Locks~

There isn't a foxette alive who doesn't know the meaning of "bad hair day." But a few tips can help shorten your routine—and save you from a headache or two.

• Your routine should start with a shampoo and conditioner to suit your hair type, followed by a cold-water rinse to seal hair cuticles and add shine. To cut down on drying time, wrap hair in a fast-absorbing towel while you do your makeup. Then unwrap and let your hair air-dry as you get dressed. The less time you spend under a blow-dryer, the less damage. Use a wide-tooth comb and natural bristle brush to prevent breakage. And who can resist a little extra glossing serum or cream to help defrizz, deflate, and foxify.

Foxy Time-Saver: Leave-in conditioners save valuable seconds when you're combing out your hair. They detangle, smooth, and condition all in one.

• To preserve a salon or at-home blow out, and give your hair a rest, you don't have to wash it every day. The oils in your hair make it easier to work with and act as a natural conditioner. Going more than a day without washing your hair also saves time and damage from daily blow-drying. This even works for fine hair—give it a whirl!

Foxy Time-Saver: If you have medium-length or long hair, sleep with it tied in a loose "Pebbles Flintstone-style" ponytail or a bun on top of your head. This will help keep it from getting too wild overnight. In the A.M., shake and comb it out, rub smoothing serum throughout, and give it a quick blast with the hair dryer. Finish off with a few shots of a glossing hair spray.

• Don't frump out with faded color. Whether you color your hair at a salon or at home, try to keep it up.
• Don't wait for pesky grays to pop out, or dark roots to spread like wildfire. Salon color can be pricey, but it's worth it—and the chances of coming out with green hair are pretty slim.

Foxy Time-Saver: Color-hued shampoos and conditioners will extend the life of your color in between salon visits.

• Foxy Short Hair: Use a smoothing hair gel or molding cream to create choppier styles. Play around with a headband or small barrettes to create your own look.
• Foxy Medium Hair: Use a volumizer and a large round natural bristle brush to create shape. Try a headband or ponytail when you're not in the mood to labor over your locks.
• Foxy Long Hair: A jumbo round or paddle brush is best for styling longer hair. They cover more area and cut down drying time. Finish with gloss or smoothing cream to tame frizzies and split ends. Or just twist it up into a tortoise shell barrel clip when it's not behaving.

Foxy Tip: A deep side part instantly gives any hair a sassy and sexy look.

~Foxy Fashion~

Now that your hair and face are foxified, it's time for a few fashion basics. We foxettes don't have many rules in life, but when it comes to clothes, our mantra is Alluring, Affordable, Adaptable.

• **Alluring.** You want clothes that look great on you. Opt for classic styles and separates that you can mix and match. Part of the allure is how you put things together (effortlessly!), and how you accessorize. Beware of fads: Leg warmers with miniskirts may dazzle on the runway, but that's where they should stay.

• **Affordable.** A little can go a long way when it comes to clothing. If you start with the right basics and tailor them to your own lifestyle, you'll never again have one of those mornings when you open up your closet full of clothes and say "I have nothing to wear." And you won't have to spend a small fortune on new pieces every season.

Foxy Tip: Spend a little extra on leather bags, jewelry, cashmere sweaters, and dress shoes. Save on flip-flops, sneakers, T-shirts, and summer clothing. Warm-weather wear is more disposable and lightweight, while cool-weather clothing tends to be heavier and more richly textured, so it can cost a bit more for quality.

• **Adaptable.** Choose clothes that play double roles in your dual life. Often you have to dash from work to an evening affair, or from the gym to lunch with friends, so make sure your outfit can carry you through.

Those are the three keys for foxettes who want to get straight A's in style. The fourth and final A is Absolutely Foxy Fit. We foxettes come in all shapes and sizes, so we try to stick with the cuts that look best on us. As much as you may love that cleavage-baring wrap top on your voluptuous friend, you might find that on you it flattens instead of flatters. To avoid frumpy fits, here are a few guidelines:

• **Small Breasts.** Flaunt what you've got, even if you haven't got a lot. Wear body-contouring silhouettes that accentuate your torso. Look for stretchy fabrics, gathered bustlines, and criss-cross tops that give your breasts added shape. Opt for three-quarter-sleeve waist-length pullovers, '50s-style cardigans, and fitted zip-up hoodies. When you want a little

Top Five Frumpy Hair Problems

• **Frizzy Hair**: Use a smoothing cream mixed with thick hair gel or glossing serum.

• **Flat Hair:** Spray on some root volumizer, create lift by blow-drying upside down, and add a spritz of hair spray to maintain shape.

• **Bad Roots:** Minimize roots by parting hair in a messy zigzag.

• **Gray Hairs:** Find some eye shadow close to the color of your hair, wet it, and blend it in to camouflage those stray grays.

• **Oily Hair:** Shake talcum powder into your palms and run your hands through your hair, starting at the roots, all the way to the ends. The powder works like a dry shampoo to absorb oils. Then work some mousse into the roots for volume and use wax to create chunky pieces and texture.

want a little extra lift, try a padded bra like Victoria's Secret Body by Victoria.

• **Bountiful Breasts.** Flatter what you've got, even if you've got a lot. Stick with anything that wraps around your upper body—dresses, belted cardigan sweaters, and jackets. Wrap styles accentuate the waist and define your breasts. Deep V-neck blazers do the same. Since short-waisted T-shirts will cut off your torso and magnify the size and width of your chest, go for longer, hip-length tees.

• **No Booty.** Define what you've got, don't drown it. You'll lose your shape in baggy bottoms, so stick with low-waist, straight-leg pants, long or cropped. Fortunately, jean companies have caught on and are designing jeans to flatter the backside. Look for styles with smaller back pockets placed higher up for the illusion of a fuller bottom. Avoid low, over-sized pockets; they just drag your tush down. Pencil and A-line skirts also help create curves.

• **Big Booty.** Treat your extra padding as a plus, not a pain in the you-know-what. Wide-leg pants that sit low on the hip minimize your backside by elongating and creating proportion. Make sure pants don't pull or pucker across your bottom. Thicker fabrics tend to hold their shape better and help conceal. Flared above-the-knee skirts lengthen your legs and minimize your rear. And hip-length jackets give you a little added coverage when you want to camouflage your shapely self.

• **Too Tall.** Embrace your height, don't hide it. Stick with styles that sit on the hip, since high-waist pants can make your legs look twice as long. Fabrics with horizontal stripes help minimize height; a striped cap-sleeve tee or boatneck sweater will draw attention to your upper bod. We don't consider long legs a problem—what could be foxier! But when you do want to shorten your leg line a bit, shoes with ankle straps will help do the job.

• **Short Legs.** Make everything south of your belly button look longer and leaner. If you want to add height, the easiest trick in the book is high heels. Go as high as you can, and stick with a longer pant to further elongate your lower bod. When wearing flats, choose something with a bit of a mini-wedge or lift, even on sneakers and flip-flops. Look for a knee-length skirt or one that hits slightly above the knee. Revealing those lovely calves will make your legs appear longer.

• **No Curves.** Create foxy curves out of straight lines. Add definition by sticking with dresses that are tapered at the waist, or try wearing a loose chain belt over your favorite drapey dress. Pants should be boot-cut style with a low waist; you'll get lost in anything too roomy. Stick with belted coats and jackets to taper your waist—or give you one.

• **Curvy.** Go fitted, rather than full and fluffy. Clothes that are too roomy won't flatter your foxy figure. Go for dark colors and smaller patterns to minimize. Opt for drawstring skirts and pants instead of elastic. Drawstring styles can sit lower on your hips and won't cut into you the way elastic does. Don't tuck in shirts; leaving them loose will lengthen your look and whittle your middle. Choose hip-length tops with a bit of a flare at the bottom; tunic and ruched styles tend to camouflage curves.

• **Hippy.** Balance your bottom, don't balloon it. Opt for wide-leg palazzo pants, since the fuller cut will reproportion your sexy silhouette. Stick with pants without back pockets, since they'll only draw attention. Dark colors always help to conceal and minimize. A-line skirts and dresses downplay your girly hips, while V-necks elongate and draw the eye to the upper bod. Three-quarter-length coats flatter almost any foxy shape, but especially curvier ones.

• **Heavy Arms.** Stick with sleeves that enhance, not enlarge. Bell sleeves add a mod touch and taper the width of your arms for a long, graceful line. Tees and blouses with three-quarter sleeves conceal any extra bulk at the back of your arms. And V-necks draw attention to your comely cleavage, and away from your arms. Shawls are an eternally foxy accessory that provide extra coverage over sleeveless tops or spaghetti-strap dresses.

• **Tailor Made.** Whether you're full figured or flat, your greatest ally in getting foxified is a good tailor. You may have found an unbelievable wool coat buried in the twenty dollar rack, but chances are it needs a little nip and tuck. Even so, it's still a bargain! You can also give new life to old clothes by having a tailor whip them up into a new cut—just like that, an outdated full-length skirt can be transformed into a stylish modern A-line.

No matter how well your clothes fit, you can't very well be foxy if you look like a patchwork quilt. Every foxy woman should know a few basics of color, texture, and pattern in order to put together the ultimate wardrobe.

~Color Me Foxy~

Foxettes know what colors they feel comfortable and sexy in. Stick with shades that work with your skin tone and hair color and that don't wash you out. Of course, you want shades that also make you feel good! Black and white are classics that work on everyone and can be mixed and matched with every color under the sun. If you're on a budget but are tempted to indulge on a high-ticket item, stick with a timeless color—not a pricey metallic bag that you'll use for only one season. Save color for your accessories, including shoes, bags, jewelry, scarves, and jackets. Try a turquoise necklace, lime green sandals, or an orange woven leather bag for a hint of tint.

~Tantalizing Textures~

Too much of a good thing isn't always good. If you're wearing jeans, choose a jacket that's twill or corduroy instead of denim. If you're wearing a suede skirt, go with leather shoes or boots, instead of more suede. If you're wearing an embroidered coat, an unembellished dress or skirt is best. You get the drift.

~Playful Patterns~

Foxettes love to play with pattern, but again, don't overdose on one theme, whether it's stripes, polka dots, paisley, or animal prints. If you're wearing a flowered skirt, stick with a solid shirt. Combine a zebra-print blouse with a solid black bottom. Go with smaller patterns such as microstripes, mini polka dots, or herringbone to downplay body parts that you're looking to minimize. Stripes can add kick, but follow this Foxy Formula: In general, stick with horizontal stripes on top and vertical on bottom, with the exception of pin-striped shirts (but please don't wear stripes on top and bottom at the same time, regardless of what direction they're going in!).

~The Basic Foxy Wardrobe~

• **T-Shirts.** T-shirts are an essential part of every foxy girl's wardrobe. They go with everything from jeans to swirly skirts, come in every color of the rainbow, and are comfy beyond compare.

- Layering tees is a look we foxettes love. The underneath layer should be thin and can be a little longer than the top layer to create a funky peek of color. Pair a camisole-style tank under a long-sleeve tee, or a long sleeve under a short sleeve.
- Experiment with color combinations like navy and pale pink, or white and yellow.
- Look for an elongated shape in tees, not a boxy shape. Tees that hit mid-hip are most flattering. And look for cotton tees with a bit of stretch to hug your lovable and lovely curves.

• **Undies.** Nothing's foxier than the right pair of panties. Keep a good stash of your favorites in black, white, and nude. We love thongs because you'll never have to worry about crunching and bunching. And keep a special pack of undies for that time of the month, so the rest will stay fresh. Foxy takes on a whole new meaning with Cosabella mesh thongs. They're so thin you can't even feel them, and they never show through clothes—an all-star in the battle against VPL (Visible Panty Lines)!

• **Bras.** Only the best for your foxy chest. A bra should fit properly, so don't go for form over function. You want bras with support *and* style. Create a bra wardrobe: a push-up or padded for dates or evenings out; full coverage for work and everyday; and a convertible bra that can switch to strapless or racerback. Foxy favorites include Victoria's Secret Body by Victoria, Warners' Fit to Be Tried, and Frederick's of Hollywood for some sizzle.

• **Hose.** We're big fans of going bare legged. If you follow our foxy tips, your legs will look sleek and you can go stockingless practically year-round. Good moisturizer and a coat of self-tanner are like your very own pair of natural stockings. But for those who aren't comfortable baring it all, or live in cold climates, choose the sheerest and most invisible pair of hose you can find. Note to self: Hose with open-toe shoes are a foxy no-no!

- Wear sheer neutral hose with shift dresses and thin mid-heel leather pumps.
- Wear sheer black hose at night with dark-colored dresses and skirts, or with dark black-tie attire.
- Wear opaque black tights with knee-length skirts and tall black boots.
- Wear fishnets with vintage-style dresses and ankle-strap shoes, or pencil skirts and pumps.

~Belts~

Belts can be tricky—too thin and it looks like you have a shoelace tied around your waist, too thick and you look like a pro wrestler. Foxettes tend to be minimalists when it comes to belts because they add bulk to your waistline, and who needs that? But there are occasions when a good belt can enhance your outfit. Every foxy girl's closet should include a two-inch-wide brown leather belt with a medium-sized embossed or western-style buckle—ultra foxy with a slightly faded pair of jeans. A thin black leather belt, white belt, and silver or gold chain belt to wear over dresses and skirts are all you need to mix and match with your foxy fashions.

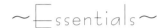

~Essentials~

Foxettes fill their closets with these must-haves to create a wardrobe that works for them, rather than a wardrobe they have to work at.

- **Black Pant Suit:** Wear with a blouse for work, a cami for dinner, or a stretchy tee.
- **White Pant Suit:** Throw on a silk tank and some gold jewelry and you're done.
- **Flat-Front Bootleg Pants:** Three or four pairs in black, white, tan, navy, or pinstripe.
- **Flared Dress Pants:** One or two pairs in silk or gabardine in cream and black.
- **Capri or Cargo Pants:** Several pairs in a style that suits your figure.
- **Jeans:** Three pairs—dark-wash straight leg for nights out, medium-wash fitted bootleg for casual everyday, and relaxed fit for weekends.
- **Leather or Suede Jacket:** A fitted hip-length style in brown, black, or wine.
- **Tees:** A variety of long- and short-sleeve tees and tanks to wear solo or layered.
- **Tailored Button-Downs:** Three-quarter and long-sleeve cotton or Lycra stretch blouses in black, white, beige, light blue, and pinstripe.
- **Cashmere Sweater Sets:** Hip-length in assorted colors like watermelon, periwinkle, sand, berry, black, and espresso.
- **Turtlenecks:** Body contouring, hip-length, in wool, cotton, or cashmere.
- **Knee-Length Skirts:** A-line, cotton drawstring, denim, flowing chiffon, wool, or gabardine pencil skirts can do no wrong. They forgive the bulges and show off your luscious legs.
- **Flared Workout Pants:** In dark colors, they'll take you from workout to weekend.
- **Zip-Up Hoodie and Wide-Leg Warm-Up Suit:** The ultimate in foxy weekend wear.
- **Wool Coat:** Single-breasted shin-length with or without a belt is the most classic.
- **Dresses:** One or two drapey cocktail dresses in black or your favorite hue, along with sundresses, wrap dresses, and shifts.
- **Shoes:** We could go on and on! A foxette can never have too many—dabble with ballet flats, sneakers, leather slingbacks, suede pumps, black leather knee boots, low ankle boots, open-toe sandals, wedges, driving loafers, and the ultimate hall-of-fame shoe . . . flip-flops!
- **Jackets:** Corduroy, jean, twill, boucle, and wool blend.
- **Handbags:** Like shoes, it's hard to have too many. Every foxette should own a structured black leather tote, an everyday shoulder bag, seasonal colored bags, and beaded evening clutches in cream and black.

So now that we've covered the basics, let's get started. We've laid things out by occasion since that's the way we foxettes dress in real life. From workouts to weddings, dates to dinner parties, we've created easy-to-use formulas designed to help simplify and stylize. In each case, there's frumpy—things we highly recommend you avoid—and foxy—things we know will light up your look. What could be simpler?

Now on to the really good stuff . . . let the foxifying begin!

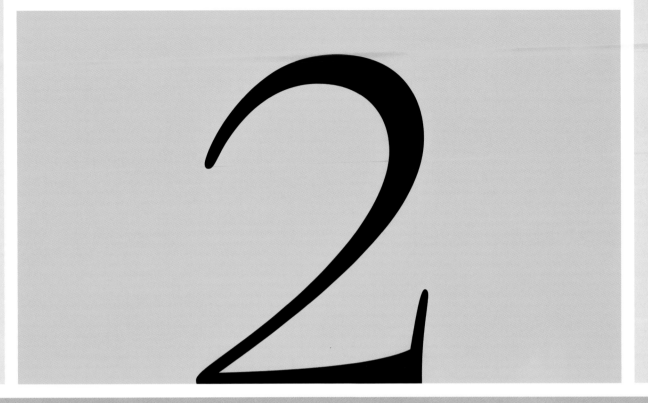

2

Foxy @ Work

Frumpy to Foxy :

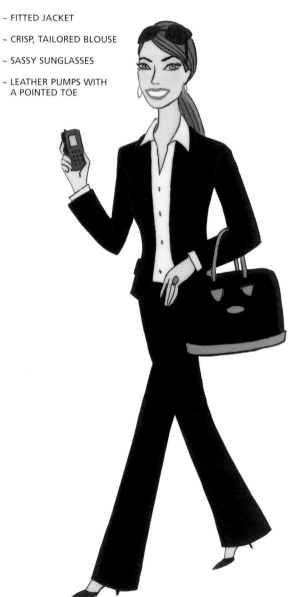

Foxy Professional

~ FITTED JACKET

~ CRISP, TAILORED BLOUSE

~ SASSY SUNGLASSES

~ LEATHER PUMPS WITH
  A POINTED TOE

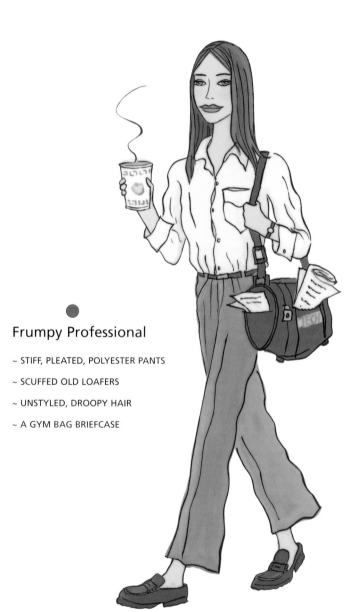

Frumpy Professional

~ STIFF, PLEATED, POLYESTER PANTS

~ SCUFFED OLD LOAFERS

~ UNSTYLED, DROOPY HAIR

~ A GYM BAG BRIEFCASE

Professional

~Frumpy Fashion~

It takes a real woman to make dressing for work look effortless. It's hard to pull that off five days a week—especially when your alarm clock blares at 6:00 A.M. and you're shuffling bleary-eyed into your regimen of showering, hair curling, makeup plastering, shirt ironing, dog feeding, newspaper reading, coffee chugging, and car pooling. It's no surprise that the daily grind can get you into a fashion rut.

Those stiff and starchy pleated polyester pants that are an inch too short may be your "comfy work pants," but they need to go into retirement. And the plain Jane white blouse that's yellowing around the neck would never get the boss's stamp of approval. Neither would those scuffed-up old loafers that have been walking you to and from the office daily for the last five years. You may have to commute, but your outfit shouldn't look like it has extra mileage.

Skirts make for a polished office look, but a full-length pleated-style skirt coupled with an oversized blouse looks like the uniform of a prep school matron. On the other hand, a super-high suede miniskirt is way too sexy for the workplace. If you can't sit cross-legged at your desk without showing a little panty, then it's not foxy-certified "work wear." And on a similar note: No one at work wants to see your nipples in all their glory. You may be doing your job, but that flimsy bra isn't doing its!

Working women understand that a day-to-day work bag has to be practical and roomy, and as much as you love two-for-one bargains, your gym bag shouldn't double as a briefcase. You may have just come from your 7:00 A.M. step class (kudos), but do all your coworkers have to know?

~Frumpy Face and Bod~

Who doesn't want to smell good at work? But stay away from overpowering "old lady" scents. You don't want your coworkers to smell you before they see you and run hiding into the copy room to avoid getting poofed by your perfume.

And while there is always some place in the world for flowered, striped, and bedazzled nails, it's not the office.

Frumpy to Foxy in 15 Minutes

~Foxy Fashion~

No matter what path your career takes, make sure you punch in looking like a pro.

The core of any working girl's wardrobe is a beautiful black suit. The possibilities are endless: It goes with every color, looks good on every body shape, and minimizes faults. And it's the most versatile piece of clothing under the sun. Choose one that's modern but won't be out of style in a year. Look for a fitted jacket that hits mid-hip and has a little stretch. Pants should be long and flared to elongate your bod; hem them at least one-half inch longer than usual and wear them with heels for a look that is sleek and chic.

Foxy Tip: Men have a good eye for how suits should fit, so take a guy along when you try them on.

We'd never make it through a week of meetings and office mania without a classic shift dress to keep us looking cool. Again, basic black is the ticket. Wear it alone in the summer with a pair of mid-heel slides, which are more suitable for work than a strappy sandal, or mix it with a colorful cardigan and a pair of knee-high leather boots in the winter.

Round out your week with a few foxy essentials. Sassy knee-length pencil skirts in rich colors like reds, plums, wines, and dark blues blend in with the sophisticated feel of the professional office. Stock up on tailored long-sleeve blouses, including a crisp white one (with French cuffs for extra class), plus a handful of silk camisoles for layering and a supportive bra. For the changing seasons, toss in a few hip-length wool blend turtlenecks and cotton or cashmere crewneck sweater sets.

Foxy Tip: Since you make your office clothes work as hard as you do, don't be shy about retiring items when they lose their luster. Chuck blouses if they start to yellow around the neck or underarms.

As you strut your stuff around the office, shoe choices are easy. Unless you're going for a vintage look, a shapely pair of black pumps with a pointed toe is more flattering than rounded. Knee-high black boots are ultra-versatile—you can wear them with skirts and bootleg pants. And a mid-heel pair of wedge sandals creates a foxy casual look that goes with anything and won't leave you wobbling on your way to the water cooler like a pair of stiletto heels might. Foxettes also like peep-toe heels; they keep our feet covered with just enough pretty polished toe peeking out. Don't be afraid to experiment with color. Wear a pair of red heels to punch up a black suit, or spice up a chocolate brown skirt with light pink mules.

Foxy Tip: We clock in a lot of mileage on our work shoes. The easiest way to keep them from looking frumpy is to treat them to an occasional polish. To get the most out of an expensive pair of shoes, find a good repair shop—they can make a five-year-old shoe look brand new.

Look divine from desk to business dinner with a few classic accessories: a works-with-everything medium-size stainless steel watch, silver or pearl dangle earrings, a colorful silk scarf for drizzly dreary days, and sassy sunglasses for sunny ones. You can mix and match these basics with colorful chokers, artsy coral rings, and other goodies, but these are the essentials that make dressing every day easy and foxy.

One of the toughest things about foxy work-day dressing is that you're often headed somewhere right after work, so you need outfits and bags that will transition. That's why the Big Black Tote in nylon or soft buttery leather is the ultimate creation. You can lug stuff to work and unload it into your desk, then use the bag throughout the day as a briefcase. After work, load your goodies back in and hit the road.

With this savvy and stylish set of items, you can foxify Monday through Friday. And you'll look so effortless, no one will ever know you're working it, working girl!

~Foxy Hair~

If dressing for work five days a week is hard, figuring out what to do with that unruly hair can be even tougher. Since you have to do this beauty ritual five days a week, usually before you've had that first eye-opening cup o' joe, simple is better.

For a fuss-free professional style, smooth out long or medium hair with glossing serum and pull it back into a ponytail with a snag-free black elastic band. For short hair, try a thin, stretchy headband.

~Foxy Face~ and Bod

Face the day with the Foxy Five. Good lip colors for work are pinkish browns, sheer warm reds, and earthy peaches.

Nail color should be very sheer and subdued, such as an opalescent pale pink or sheer beige.

Be kind to your coworkers by sticking with subtle scents. Light citrus, ultra-sheer florals, or soft powdery fragrances are sure to earn rave reviews.

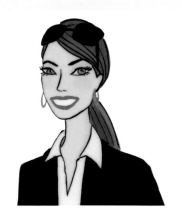

Frumpy to Foxy:

~Frumpy Fashion~

Because California career foxettes appreciate the relaxed style that warmer weather offers, they provide a perfect model for casual work wear. In the land of seemingly endless sunshine, you can go for days in short-sleeve T-shirts, cotton skirts, and slides. But things can get sticky when you take your look for granted and fall into a frump trap.

Even if you live near a body of water, it's best to steer away from vacation-style clothing such as sundresses or Hawaiian print blouses with Bermuda shorts. The goal is to look clean and career oriented, not "cowabunga!"

You'll really be pushing it by sliding into rubber flip-flops. The laid-back style of the casual office can make it tempting, but in order to avoid getting stuck low down on the corporate ladder, stash them away until Saturday.

While jeans are a staple in casual offices, nix the ones that are bleached out and torn from years of wash and wear, or almost transparent from frequent trips to the dryer. When you confidently stride into the conference room and take a seat at the weekly executive meeting, the last thing you want everyone to hear is "rrrrrrrrip!" Also, avoid any jeans with lots of detailing. Save the fringe and beading for your next trip to the rodeo, cowgirl.

Unfortunately, homework didn't end when you kissed your final day of school good-bye. During the week, you may need extra gear to carry all those documents and reading materials home. Rather than traipsing into the office with two overstuffed bags with papers sticking out every which way, opt for one large style with several compartments to keep everything organized. You don't want the boss to think you're out to lunch when you aren't!

Casual

Foxy Casual

~ JERSEY DRAWSTRING SKIRT

~ FITTED T-SHIRT

~ PALE PINK LIP GLOSS

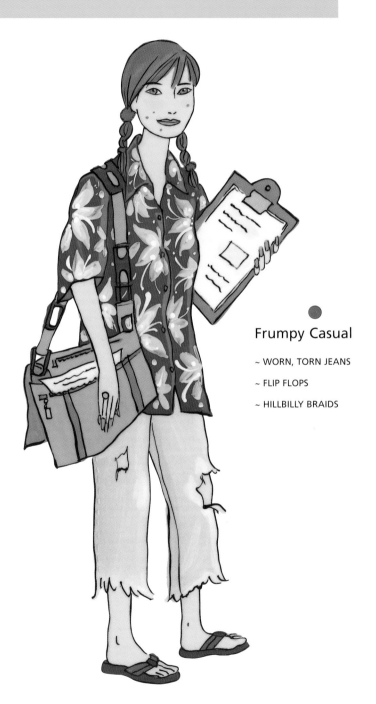

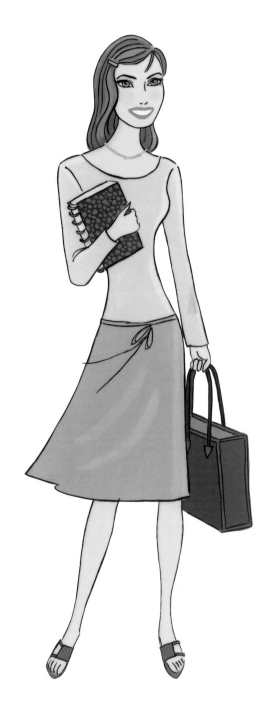

Frumpy Casual

~ WORN, TORN JEANS

~ FLIP FLOPS

~ HILLBILLY BRAIDS

And, even though they're a must for an outdoor break on a bright, sunny day, hats seem a bit silly inside the office. Sure, casual work style can be relaxed, but this is the office, not the great outdoors. Wearing your baseball cap into the conference room will not help you score a home run—or that big bonus.

~Frumpy Face and Bod~

Looking professional at work isn't just about a winning outfit. Hair and makeup are also key players on the team. Messy dos have no place in the office, so keep it casual and carefree, yet combed. Braids are fine for the weekend, but may look a little too hillbilly for the office, so save them for your day off.

Sadly, just like homework, breakouts also haven't ended just because you're no longer a teen. If tight deadlines have been making you feel stressed for weeks and your face is taking it out on you, there's a good chance those pesky pimples could start popping up. Not the best time to frump out, and those fluorescent office lights don't help matters.

~Foxy Fashion~

See you at the top, Foxy! Maintaining casual elegance Monday through Friday can be a breeze. And, what more could you want than not having to fret over what to wear five days a week!

For a polished and professional look, foxettes stock up on knee-length jersey or cotton skirts with an elastic or drawstring waist. They're comfortable and forgiving, especially when you're sitting in front of a computer for hours after a heavy lunch. Paired with a button-down Lycra shirt or a colorful T-shirt and open-toe slides, this look can take you straight from meetings with coworkers to cocktails with friends. Slides are the working girl's answer to flip-flops; they're comfy yet not too casual. It can't hurt to have a pair in basic black and classic brown. And for those days when you want to add a little color, try a pair in red.

Foxy in 15 Minutes

Beige or black lightweight bootleg slacks in stretchy wool or cotton are another cherished staple. They have just the right amount of give and don't wrinkle like linen. If it's extra warm, you can't beat seersucker; it's lightweight and never goes out of style. Steer away from pleats. The smooth-front styles are much more becoming, and when you sit down, they won't puff out and make you look like you have a pillow stuck down there. Round the look out with a button-down waist-length cardigan sweater or a funnel-neck, sleeveless knit top, and leather peep-toe heels. You'll look so smart, everyone will know who's on her way up that ladder.

When we think of the casual office, we think of jeans. Stick with a more refined, darker wash that doesn't ride too low on the hips. The last thing you want is to give your coworkers a peek at your hot-pink panties. To polish off this casual look with the flair of a pro, add a stretchy crew-neck T-shirt, a hip-length, single-breasted, tailored jacket, and leather slingbacks to show them who's in charge.

Many career foxettes prefer to go stockingless—blame it on the weather! When it's just too cold for bare legs, reach for sheer black or nude hose.

If you want to keep things easy, a medium-size canvas or leather tote should fit all of your personal belongings as well as those top-secret documents. On those days when you have a lot of extra "homework," your everyday bucket bag along with a roomy carryall will do the trick.

~Foxy Hair~

Keep your foxy head high, and you could be running the show in no time!

When your hair isn't cooperating and you're pestered by annoying wisps that won't stay in place, clip them back with small barrettes. This can work for any length hair; the key is to match them to the color of your hair so they blend in. For some reason, the workday seems that much more manageable when your tresses are performing well.

~Foxy Face and Bod~

As for your nine-to-five face, once again it's the Foxy Five. It'll make that morning rush hour less of a rush.

Your boss may think you're a breakout talent, but when you need to hide a big red bump on your face, use a heavy-duty cover-up. Oxy makes a cover-up with zit zapper—that means double duty. If only office politics were that easy!

For those foxy nails, brush on a coat of something sheer. A soft pink or sweet, pale lavender will do the trick.

Frumpy to Foxy:

Frumpy Job Interview

~ WRINKLED BLOUSE

~ DARK, VAMPY NAIL POLISH

~ OVERSIZED "LOGO" BAG

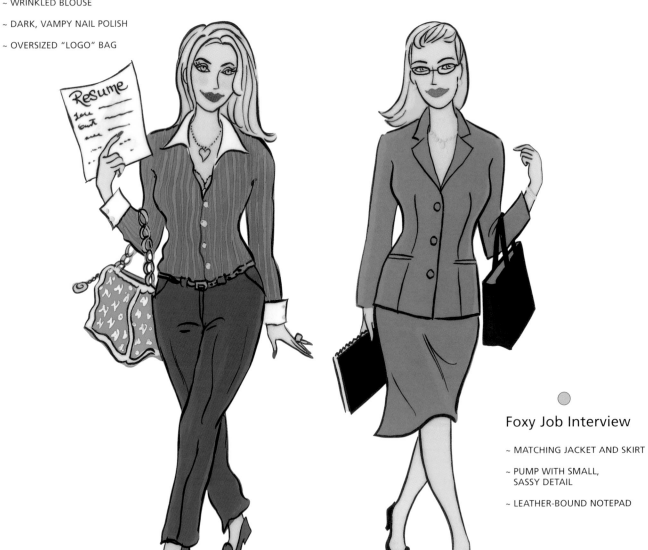

Foxy Job Interview

~ MATCHING JACKET AND SKIRT

~ PUMP WITH SMALL, SASSY DETAIL

~ LEATHER-BOUND NOTEPAD

Job Interview

~Frumpy Fashion~

You've spent the last twenty-four hours rehearsing why you're the best candidate for the job. "I'm organized, I stay calm under pressure, and I'm a clever strategist" keeps running through your head. Almost as important is the dress rehearsal, so you mustn't forget "I'm foxy." Otherwise, one frumpy move could land you right back on the sofa with the classifieds in hand.

In addition to bowling them over with your smarts, you want to walk into your future employer's office looking like the polished and professional foxette you are. A crinkly blouse and wrinkled slacks with static cling won't make the cut. So before you head out your door, be sure to do a triple take—otherwise, the interviewer could show you the door.

While an elegant, partially off-the-shoulder sweater may look stunning, showing too much skin is not, at least at this stage. Maybe after you've worked there for a couple months and shown them what you're made of, but for now, you don't want a fashion statement that says anything other than "hire me!" It's also a good idea to stay away from extra bold, bright colors like fuchsia, lime green, and electric blue. If the boss-to-be is conservative, overdosing on color the first time you meet may be distracting. The goal is to turn on their interest, not turn them off.

Strutting into your interview sporting a pair of slinky stilettos and a purse covered with poodles isn't going to help your résumé. And for this occasion, forget the oversized designer logo bag—the only name you want them to remember is yours!

~Frumpy Face and Bod~

Even if we're pretty pleased with our choice of "career girl" clothes, walking in with untamed hair and heavy makeup won't please the powers that be. You're trying to get the job, not get ready for a Halloween party. Job interviews can give you a jumbo case of the jitters, but a face full of the frumps is no way to get ahead.

Make sure to impress potential employers with common sense, not scents. Your friends may love your strong, floral perfume, but that doesn't mean the future boss will. While you share your long list of qualifications, the blast of bouquet may leave your would-be employer focusing on how to get you to stop wearing it instead of recognizing how competent you are. Funky nail polish in deep, vampy colors can almost look black in an office that isn't well lit. As stylish as dark polish can be, a potential employer may not agree. With fingers like that, who cares how many words a minute you can type!

Frumpy to Foxy in 15 Minutes 🕐

~Foxy Fashion~

Nail it, Foxy! Glide into that office looking like a million bucks and let them know you're the only candidate for the job!

Nothing says "I'm the one" like a matching jacket and knee-length skirt in tweed, bouclé fabric. Stick with colors such as brown, navy blue, or black; subtle pastels work well, too, in the spring and summer. You don't even need to wear a shirt underneath—just keep the jacket buttoned up enough to cover your bra, and you'll prove that you're buttoned up as well.

If your dream job is with a conservative company, cover your gams with very sheer nude hose and walk tall in two-inch leather pumps with a slightly pointed toe. Instead of a plain shoe, choose one with unique detailing like a tiny bow, carved heel, or decorative stitching to show your prospective new employer that you're sensible and stylish, but not stuffy.

Dark, flared wool-blend slacks will also do the job. Pair them with a coordinating jacket and a crisp, white button-down shirt with high-heel brown or black loafers and you're sure to impress—who needs references! Just remember that dark colors love to attract lint and other fuzzies, so make sure to do a 360-degree check before heading out the door. Always keep a lint roller handy for a once-over, especially if you've been snuggling with your furry friends, Peanut and Mr. Jinx.

Your goal, other than getting hired, is to look fuss-free and

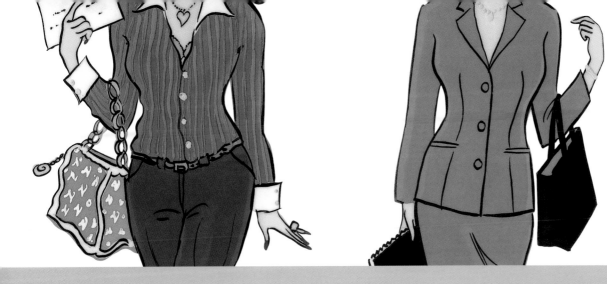

refined, so jewelry should be kept to a minimum. You don't need anything more than a couple of stackable rings, a tank-style watch, stud earrings, and a thin necklace.

The simplicity rule goes for your handbag as well. Carry a small- to medium-size tote or shoulder bag to seal the deal. Don't forget to pop a small leather-bound notepad inside to jot down questions and take notes. If you want to add some color to show off your personality without going overboard, accessorize with a solid bag in a subtle color like dark red or pale yellow—nothing that will take the attention away from you.

Now go break a leg!

~Foxy Hair~

Just like a status report, simplicity and efficiency are key when it comes to hair. Win them over by pulling your tresses all the way off your face either in a low ponytail or clipped back in a half-up/half-down do. Your bright, determined eyes should be in full view.

~Foxy Face and Bod~

If you haven't had time for a manicure, brush your nails with quick-drying, clear polish. Tidy hands will help assure them you're efficient and orderly. Close the deal with a firm handshake!

When it comes to scent, keep it subtle or don't wear anything more than a spread of fresh-scented lotion. Jergens is a flawless foxy staple. The boss (to be) will definitely approve.

Frumpy to Foxy:

~Frumpy Fashion~

What's not to love about Fridays? Not only is it the prelude to a wild and foxified weekend, but it's also the day that we working gals get to roll up our pantyhose in revolt and celebrate that fabulous phenom called Casual Fridays. Yet while we love any excuse to dress comfy, we've also seen Casual Fridays go dreadfully wrong.

Resist the urge to turn Casual Friday into Frumpy Friday. This is not an excuse for you to pull out your faded jeans and saggy seen-better-days sweaters. Jeans are popular Friday office attire, but if they're done wrong, you can go from Calvin Klein poster girl to frumpy farm girl in a heartbeat. No true foxy girl would show up at work looking like she's dressed for a day of yard work; you always want to dress to impress.

Jeans are a great Friday option, but stay away from baggy styles. They look more careless than casual, and they definitely don't get across that "denim chic" look you're trying to achieve. Nor do those well-worn flannel shirts; save them for the campground. Golf shirts work on the golf course, not in the board room. And those T-shirts bearing company logos and silly slogans (KISS ME I'M IRISH) will come off as sloppy, not savvy. For those searingly hot summer Fridays, shorts may be tempting but are a big no-no at the office.

Casual doesn't mean sneakers—sorry, never at work, foxettes. Leave the running shoes for running and the loafers for loafing. Bottom line: Anything suitable for jogging, hiking, or mud-wrestling won't cut it. We working girls gotta work it, girl—from head to glorious toe.

~Frumpy Face and Bod~

Maybe it's been a long week and you're feeling too lazy for your own good, but coming to work with freshly shampooed, still-wet hair isn't going to help a foxy girl climb that corporate ladder. You'll only end up looking soggy instead of successful.

Alas, Casual Friday doesn't mean we can clock in wearing no makeup and yesterday's dingy hairdo. A sloppy, lumpy ponytail that you didn't comb out and missing makeup are going to make your coworkers wonder if you stayed out too late partying the night before. Wonder what the boss would think . . .

Sometimes our zeal over the impending weekend makes us a bit too eager to bring weekend habits into the workplace, but grooming is a seven-days-a-week essential, so we can't let our look slip just because the clock's ticking toward five o'clock.

Fridays

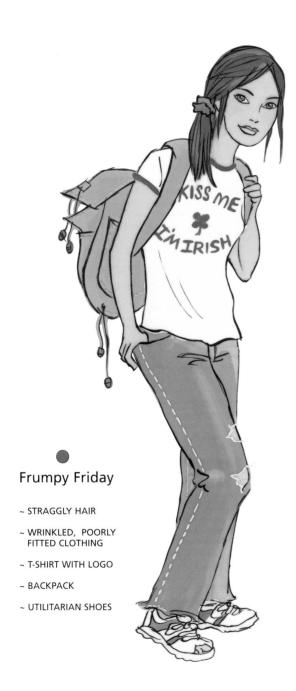

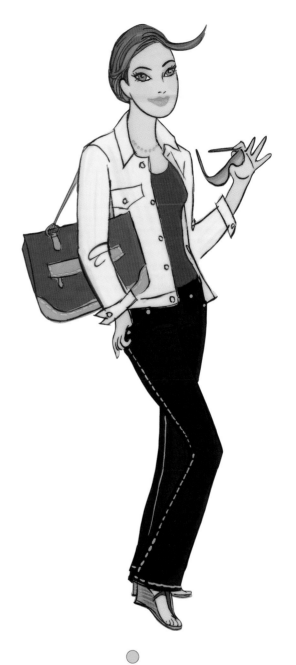

Frumpy Friday

~ STRAGGLY HAIR

~ WRINKLED, POORLY FITTED CLOTHING

~ T-SHIRT WITH LOGO

~ BACKPACK

~ UTILITARIAN SHOES

Foxy Friday

~ DARK JEANS

~ COLORED T-SHIRT

~ NEAT MATCHING BAG

~ WEDGE SANDALS

~ SIMPLE, ELEGANT JEWELRY

~Foxy Fashion~

Now that's the way to work it, foxy girl! Dress for foxy success, even on Fridays.

One of our favorite foxy Friday looks is a sleek pair of dark jeans—fitted but not hiney-huggin'—along with a contoured tee and short, shaped jacket. We love corduroy or stretchy gabardine jackets since texture adds oomph to the outfit. If your T-shirt is colored, try a more neutral jacket—and vice versa—so your look has some depth. In cooler weather, replace the tee with a body-hugging cashmere hip-length turtleneck. It's the foxette's winter version of a T-shirt. The added bonus: These looks transition seamlessly to after-work happy hour.

Another foxy Friday option: Start with cotton capris, which are an office-appropriate alternative to shorts when things heat up. Wear them with a tank and cotton zip-up cardigan or a classic three-quarter-sleeve blouse, and you're ready to roll. When the AC is blasting, it's nice to have your arms covered up.

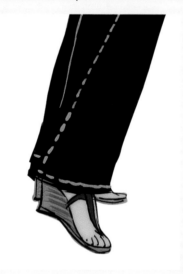

As for those nine-to-five feet, deck them out in wedge sandals, ankle boots, or girly flats. All are clever but comfy choices that don't look too casual or carefree. The people you work with—and for—will give you bonus points for making Fridays fabulously foxy.

Foxy Fridays are also a good time to have fun with accessories. Whimsical beaded earrings, a colorful oversized watch, or funky charm bracelet can be the ideal "let loose" accent to top it all off. It's the perfect way to show the staff your personality without looking unprofessional.

Replace the briefcase with a relaxed suede or nylon tote that will fit your papers and any other extracurricular stuff you need to take home over the weekend. It'll also be roomy enough to fit those few extras that a foxette needs to get ready for the Friday night festivities: shimmer eye shadow, lip gloss, and maybe even a lacy cami to replace that T-shirt.

Once you have the right fashion formula in place, all your envious coworkers will realize the true meaning of TGIF is "This Girl Is Foxy!"

~Foxy Hair~

Friday hair should be foxy as usual. If you don't have time to do a full blow out, at least give your hair a quick shot with the dryer to tame the sopping-wet look. If you have thick or long locks that take forever to air dry, work in some light gel to give them shape and twist them up into a clip. That way no one can tell your hair is damp— we foxettes are a bit sly, after all!

For stick-straight or fine hair, a glamorous high ponytail or sleek side ponytail draped over one shoulder works wonders and wins bonus points with the boss.

~Foxy Face and Bod~

Depending on what your Friday night plans are, you can tone up or tone down the Friday face.

If it's Chinese takeout and a movie marathon with the family, stick with the Foxy Five: cover up, powder, blush, mascara, and lipstick. With the casual vibe of Friday, try out a new lipstick color, such as a light wine red or bronzy beige.

If, on the other hand, you're gearing up for a night of drinks and dancing, take it up a notch. Create a good base so later on all you have to do is enhance, don your dancing shoes, and go. A light natural foundation, a dab of bronzer, light doe-y brown eye shadow, and a sweep of mascara give you a look that can go from desk to dance-floor with just a little touching up. After you clock out, pump up the volume with a sweep of shimmery beige eye shadow, a quick sweep with your eyelash curler, and a touch of rich red lipstick. Then ring in your foxy Friday night.

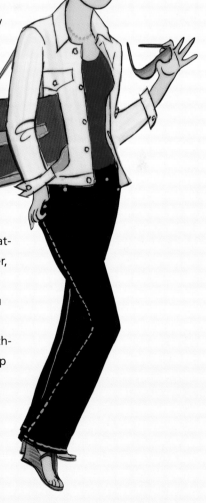

3

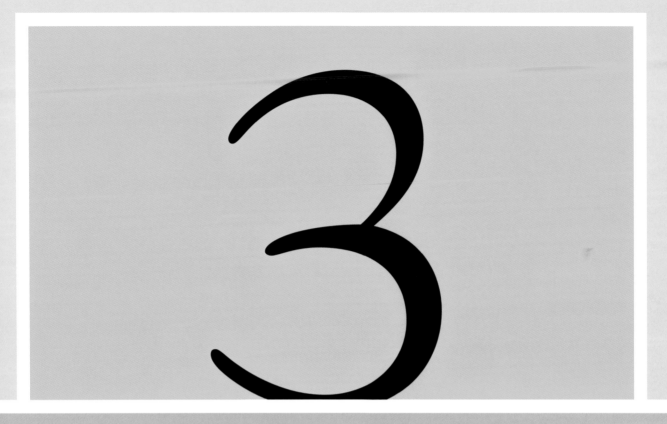

Foxy in Love

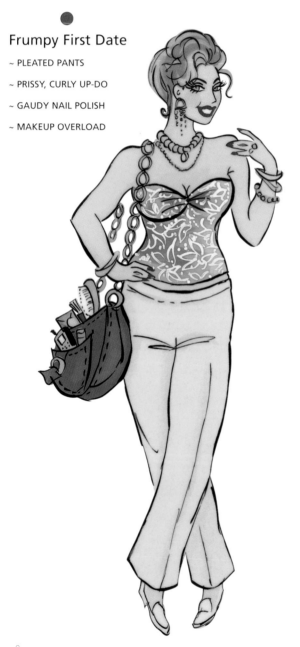

Frumpy First Date

~ PLEATED PANTS

~ PRISSY, CURLY UP-DO

~ GAUDY NAIL POLISH

~ MAKEUP OVERLOAD

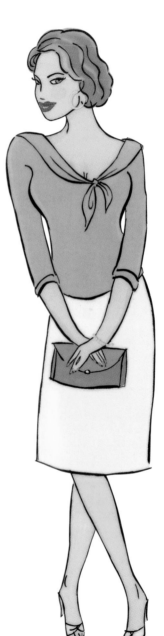

Foxy First Date

~ SWIRLY A-LINE SKIRT

~ FOXY SNAKESKIN CLUTCH

~ SEXY HOOP EARRINGS

~ VELVETY, LUSCIOUS LIPS

Date

~Frumpy Fashion~

If there's one occasion in life when every girl wants to look her foxiest, it's the First Date, the most sweat-inducing, nail-biting dressing dilemma of them all. You're nervous, you're giddy, you want to look sexy, cute, cuddly, kissable—so much pressure! A fashion faux pas can turn your first date into a frumpy fright night.

You want to be comfy on any first date, so this is not the time to wear those four-inch stilettos or that tube top that stays up only when you hold your breath. But don't take the comfort thing too far. A first date should be special, so leave the khakis and crewnecks at home.

Jeans and a T-shirt say casual and careless, so save them for the weekend, not that first "wow" date. Also steer clear of anything that adds extra bulk to your foxy frame. The worst offenders are pleated pants and long tailored blazers with NFL-approved shoulder pads; they may be good for scoring touchdowns, but not for scoring guys.

We want a beau to see us in all our girly glory, but there are certain things he *shouldn't* see on a first date. No visible panty lines. No dangling bra straps (it can look sloppy and, dare we say, even a bit too inviting). And no down-to-there cleavage. Displaying Baywatch-style breasts during the early dating stages may be too distracting and could render your hunky escort unable to absorb an ounce of what you've said over the last three hours. Plus, don't you want to give him something to explore in dates 2, 3, 4 . . . ?

Finally, we mustn't neglect dating details such as shoes and bags. Best to forgo the flats since they can look a little, well, flat. Same for shoes with a bulky square toe, since they can look boxy instead of foxy.

Resist the urge to go out on a date with the same bag you carry to work—that ten-pound potato sack stuffed with a cell phone, date book, hairbrush, lipstick, crumbs of pressed powder, gum, emergency chocolate, and other assorted girly goodies.

~Frumpy Face and Bod~

As your prince charming gazes dreamily at you all night long, you want to make sure that what he sees is fairy tale, not frumpy. No casual ponytails; save those for the gym or summer dates once he's become your steady Eddie. And no prissy curly up-dos. Guys want hair they can run their fingers through, and fussy or frizzy won't turn you into his foxy dream date.

Neither will chipped nails or gaudy nail polish, so keep them clean. Let him see *you*—don't overdo. The same goes for hairspray, jewelry, makeup, and definitely perfume, lest your date pass out in a pow of flowery fragrance. And one last tip: No rose water fragrance allowed on a first date. It reminds some guys of grandma—a sure-fire buzz-kill.

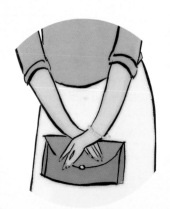

~Foxy Fashion~

Helloooo, Foxy! It's true that you never get a second chance to make a first impression, so put your all into any first date and pull out all the foxy stops. The key is to be comfy but also a knockout—to look naturally foxy, not like you spent hours fussing and prepping. Guys want a gal who looks foxy without looking like she tried. And in fifteen minutes flat, you can do just that.

If you feel sexy and sassy in pants, then greet your guy in black wool or cotton flared slacks with a slightly low waist (but no peek-a-boo thongs). Slacks like these never disappoint, and they work whether he's taking you to a romantic restaurant or an action flick. Pair them with a satiny camisole peeking out from under a brightly colored cardigan. A camisole shows off your collarbone and a hint of cleavage without diving too deep. Finish off with a choker or sexy lariat necklace to accentuate your kissable neck. Top it all off with a snakeskin clutch, and you're ready to knock him dead with all that foxiness!

If, on the other hand, you sometimes prefer the swirly, girly feel of a skirt, then an above-the-knee A-line in a fluid fabric like chiffon, rayon, or silk provides foxy flair for that first date. Wear it with a form-fitting V-neck sweater or a flirty, flutter-sleeve top in the summer; either one is romantic without being racy. The finishing touch is earrings, nothing too Cleopatra— try a sexy hoop or small dangle. Go for something with colorful beads or gemstones; the sparkle will light up your foxy face all night.

Pick a romantic color palette for those all-important first dates. Pastels can be pretty and feminine, but you don't want to overdo it and come off looking more like an Easter egg. Instead, stick with classy black or creamy beige neutrals, or set the mood with rich blush colors like dusty purples, wines, and warm bare pinks.

As for shoes, there's only one way to go on a first date—heels! A two- to three-inch-high open-toe sandal with a thin heel that slims the leg is sweet and sexy at the same time.

You've taken care of the outside, now make sure you're just as foxy underneath. A lace thong panty gives you that extra dose of allure, even if you're the only one who knows you're wearing it. Plus, it keeps unattractive panty lines at bay. Really turn things out with a matching push-up bra. He'll wonder what that playful glimmer in your eye is all about.

~Foxy Hair~

Nothing screams foxy more than a fresh new do, so this is the time to splurge on a salon blow out. Whether you go with a style that's smooth and straight, cool and curly, or fem and flippy, tresses that are soft and silky never disappoint and are essential for instant foxification. Having a pro handle your hair will take some of the pressure off—as if you don't have enough pre-date jitters!

Use silky hair spray with a slight sheen to give your locks gorgeous glow. And spray a light misting of perfume in your hair before he comes to pick you up. "Gee, your hair smells terrific" will be the first of many flattering comments he bestows throughout the night.

~Foxy Face and Bod~

For that First Date face, it's all about the lips, so play them up with lots of neutral "come hither" gloss or creamy lipstick in a deep color like raspberry red. Make sure to take that tube along for repeated applications. Foxy means velvety, luscious lips all night long that will be beckoning him for a tender first goodnight kiss.

Enhance the Foxy Five with a dash of shimmery rose powder or

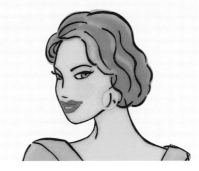

bronzer to give your cheeks a healthy flush that will make your date blush.

You want to make sure you smell as sweet as you look. Go subtle and soft with fragrance; a light musky scent or floral will attract but not overpower. Tap around your neck, behind your ears, and among your décolletage—or just spritz and walk through it for an overall burst of scent. Indulge in foxy first-date fragrances like Creative Scentualization's Perfect Veil and Tova.

We foxettes love French pedicures—if your date doesn't have a foot fetish, he'll develop one that night!

Finally, don't forget deodorant, just in case those first-date jitters get your body heat up. In the event that things go oh-so-well, you want to be able to lift your arms and give your new beau a big ol' foxy hug! *Vive l'amour!*

Frumpy Steady Date

~ PUFFY, BLOODSHOT EYES

~ OLD TANK TOP

~ OILY, UNWASHED FACE

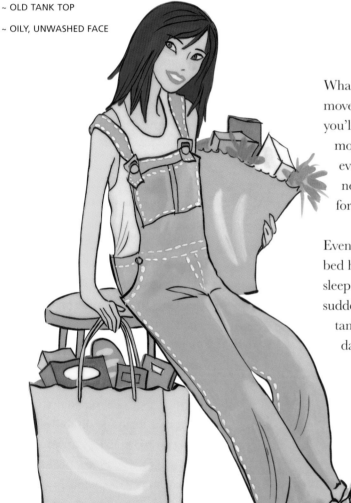

~Frumpy Fashion~

What do you know, it's on to date six and you've moved from casual dinners and wondering when you'll see each other again to steady weekends of movies, shopping for household appliances, and even a little hand holding. Ah, the comfort zone is nearing. The key, foxettes, is not to get too comfortable and wind up in the frump zone.

Even if he's seen you at 7:00 A.M. in all your glory—bed head and half-shut, puffy eyes with crusts of sleep stuck in your lashes—that doesn't mean you can suddenly stroll around in washed-out overalls with a tank top and sneakers. Don those when you take a day trip to the milk farm together.

You may be tempted to roll out of bed and straight into a shapeless gray sweat suit and plastic slides for a quick jaunt to the coffee shop. We know he'll love you anyway, but imagine how you'll feel running into his best friend—the one he's been so excited for you to meet. "Not so pleased to meet you looking like this" is what you may end up thinking.

Date

And beware of slacking off on those enduring "date nights." Ankle-length skirts paired with oversized thigh-length shirts may be appropriate for a weekend seminar or pottery class, but don't get used to wearing that little ensemble around him.

He may start wondering what happened to the foxy girl he fell for. It doesn't matter that he's seen you blow a bunch of funny goop from your nose and cough up a storm during your bout with the flu. In order to keep the romance alive, we have to keep the foxiness alive, too.

~Frumpy Face and Bod~

You've stayed home on Saturday nights to cook together, you've gone to brunch with each other's friends, and you may have even met the family. And recently he began leaving his blue toothbrush in your bathroom. The term "boyfriend" is definitely nearing.

Remember, foxettes, those clever frumps have a funny way of creeping up on you the moment you and he get close. Before you know it, you're clipping your toenails on his sofa in shapeless pajamas with dark green seaweed mask all over your face.

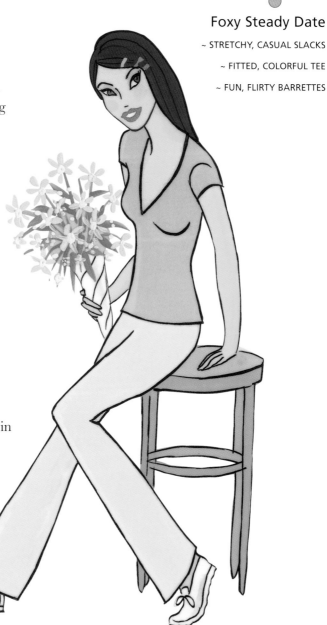

Foxy Steady Date

~ STRETCHY, CASUAL SLACKS

~ FITTED, COLORFUL TEE

~ FUN, FLIRTY BARRETTES

We're all for letting loose and cozying up together, but that's what we call going into Frumpy Overdrive. Put on the brakes!

There are always those date nights when you don't have time to freshen up before leaving work. You grab a peek in the rearview mirror to find the end-of-the-day look settled right in—flat hair, oily skin, bloodshot eyes and all. On these occasions, steer clear of restaurants with bright, fluorescent lights. He may think a dimly lit, cozy restaurant has "mood lighting," but you know it's creative camouflage!

Frumpy to Foxy in 15 Minutes

~Foxy Fashion~

Love is in the air, so keep it flowing, Foxy! Have him counting the minutes until he sees you again.

If you're still stuck on the "getting to know each other" hump and need a bit of an icebreaker, slip into a knockout number for your next romantic outing. A silky, knee-length, jewel-tone dress with spaghetti straps and strappy heels should help move things along.

On the other hand, you may be merrily coasting along together, but that doesn't mean we foxettes will let things slide. For relaxed evenings of dinner and a movie, straight-leg jeans or stretchy slacks with a '50s-inspired short-sleeve print blouse or cashmere crew neck is low-key yet still stylish. Colorful suede loafers or sleek leather ankle boots will keep him wrapped around your foxy finger.

During the colder months, besides using him to keep you warm, cover up with a thick shin-length wrap coat and a colored wool knit hat. He'll marvel at how he landed such a hot girlfriend.

For those laid-back Sunday afternoons when you sleep in and linger over the newspaper together, maintain your foxiness without looking like you're trying too hard. Cover up with a silky robe, or trade your nightie for loose drawstring pants and a tank.

If you're planning on grabbing a bite together, just throw on a zip-up cardigan and sneakers, and this look will carry you right on through, even for a shared bowl of popcorn and a snuggle session later that evening.

It's one thing to doll yourself up for a single date, but as you start to see more of each other morning, noon, and night, continue to stun your newfound flame with your foxiness—and keep him coming back for more!

~Foxy Hair~

Even if he's seen most of your best dos by now, foxettes like to keep a few surprises up their sleeves. With

If date nights run the risk of falling into the frumps, that's nothing compared to the morning after. In the beginning, waking up together can be slightly unsettling. Other than having him see you at the crack of dawn with all that natural light, there's also the matter of "morning" breath. Skipping out on a good,

minty brushing before starting the day together is a major foxy offender. If he blows you an air kiss rather than laying one on you like he usually does, you'll have a sneaking suspicion why.

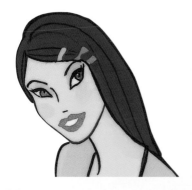

shorter hair, play it up with tiny, colorful barrettes. Clip three or four of them around the front and sides of your hair for a fresh, bubbly look. It's unexpected, just like you.

If you haven't yet worn your hair back, now's the time to give it a try. On the weekends, long ponytails can look playful and sweet. Grab one of his favorite baseball caps and pull all of your hair through the hole in the back.

Good bet he'll be thinking "home run!"

For romantic evenings out, a ponytail fastened with a silk flower elastic is sexy and sophisticated and takes less than two minutes. He'll end up spending more time on his hair than you!

~Foxy Face and Bod~

If you're meeting him for a casual dinner after a hectic day at the office that's left you looking like yesterday's blue plate special, take two minutes to powder your nose, put blush on your cheeks, comb your hair, and add a dash of lip gloss. If your eyes are bloodshot from

staring at the computer screen all day, keep a bottle of moisturizing eye drops on hand, so he can gaze into fresh, foxy eyes all evening.

When you wake up together, rather than blasting him with a dose of morning breath, take a quick jaunt to the bathroom for a rinse of mouthwash. While you're at it, revive your bedroom eyes by holding a cold, wet washcloth over them for thirty seconds to help depuff. He's not off the hook either, so don't be surprised if you find him right behind you!

Foxy Tip: Keep a packet of breath strips on the bedside table. That way, you'll get fresh breath without even having to get out of bed.

~Frumpy Fashion~

You've had a few successful dates, and he's smitten enough to show you off to his folks, or perhaps in some cases, his kids. Fellow foxettes, if he's counting on their approval to move the love-fest forward, here's where one unforgettably frumpy move could force you to do some major damage control. And fast!

If you're both ready to take this slightly nerve-racking step, then you have to play along like the foxette you are. Strolling into the restaurant with a skirt hiked up to your pelvis and a skin-tight, nipple-baring sheer T-shirt isn't going to work. Just like sexy lingerie, that enticing ensemble should be kept for naughty nights at home à deux.

Even though they're fine for certain occasions, sheer blouses are way too distracting and should be kept far away from this setting. We want his loved ones to focus on your charming self and the enlightening conversation, not your chest.

What about those platform, patent leather shoes? Sure, they can really spice things up for a night out with the girls, but you're going for refined and feminine here, not sexed out and seductive. They're more R than PG-13.

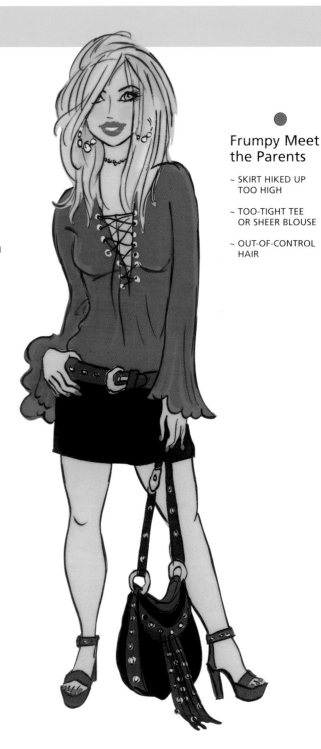

Frumpy Meet the Parents

~ SKIRT HIKED UP TOO HIGH

~ TOO-TIGHT TEE OR SHEER BLOUSE

~ OUT-OF-CONTROL HAIR

Parents (and meet the kids, too)

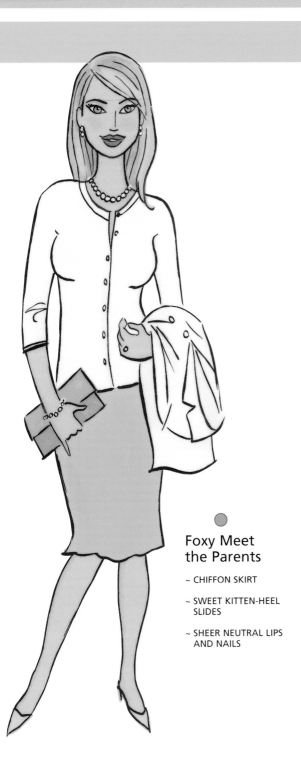

Foxy Meet the Parents

~ CHIFFON SKIRT

~ SWEET KITTEN-HEEL SLIDES

~ SHEER NEUTRAL LIPS AND NAILS

As alluring as cleavage can be, when you're deciding which bra to wear, it's wise to choose the basic everyday style with fuller coverage, not the one that catapults your bosom up and out into an entirely new dimension. Kids can be blunt and oh-so-honest, and we don't want his to blurt out "Daddy, she has such big boobs" halfway through the meal. His family may be the harshest critics you'll face, so make sure they give you two thumbs up, not two raised eyebrows.

~Frumpy Face and Bod~

As you bite into your Caesar salad, his mother will most likely be giving you another once-over through the corner of her eye. Make sure she doesn't end up fixating on a face plastered with makeup. While it's occasionally fun to punch things up by loading on the smudged, black eyeliner, the day you meet his family is not the best time to do it. The same goes for a mouth painted with gobs of thick, red, juicy lipstick. If this guy is a keeper, shouldn't a foxette pile on the charm rather than the makeup? As always, well-tamed hair is key. If it's covering your eyes and half your face, they may wonder if you have something to hide. You certainly don't want them to think you're capable of misbehaving. At least not yet!

~Foxy Fashion~

Dress to impress, Foxy! Pull out all the stops and have them wrapped around your finger. Just wait until he listens to them rave about you later on. Don't underestimate the importance of this occasion—it could pack more punch than a shot from Cupid's bow. When deciding what to wear, there's really just one way to go here: darling, demure, and debonair. Stick with colors you love, and start with a slightly loose-fitting, knee- or shin-length skirt in chiffon, rayon, or a silk blend. Fine, silky fabrics add an elegant touch. A stretchy long-sleeve cardigan sweater buttoned all the way up—so there's not an ounce of bra peeping out—is just the right complement and oh so ladylike.

Trade in those racy stilettos for sweet leather ballet flats or kitten heel slides. Pair them with a baguette purse, and his parents will greet with you with warm and inviting smiles that say "She's a keeper!"

When we're in the mood to go a bit more conservative, black pinstripe or dark solid slacks with a stretchy cotton, button-down shirt (again, not too low) and medium heel slingbacks make for a graceful entrance. Accent this look with a pearl choker and a dainty bangle bracelet.

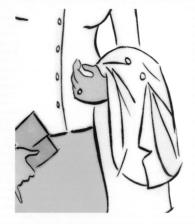

If it's cold outside, grab a sleek, shin-length wool coat or a long cardigan wrap sweater and a pair of black gloves. Of course, you can stay even warmer by nuzzling up beneath his arms.

You'll be such a hit, not only will your beau get major kudos, his parents may even invite you for brunch the following weekend. The good news is you'll know exactly what to wear!

~Foxy Hair~

This is not the time to let your hair go wild and free. You want to focus on your possible future in-laws, not that pesky chunk of hair that just won't stay in place.

For a style that looks done but not overdone, wear it half-up/half-down if your hair is long enough.

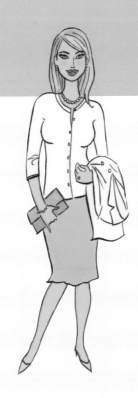

Loosely pin back the front by using small hair clips, and let a few wisps float down around the sides of your face. Go for a softer look. Stay away from a severe ponytail or slicked-back locks.

Short-hair foxettes spritz glossing spray in their locks to add extra sheen. If you can spare some Foxy Overtime, add a few soft curls with a curling iron.

~Foxy Face and Bod~

Greet his family looking like the dewy-fresh foxette you are. Depending on what his past girl-friends were like, you could have them breathing a sigh of relief the minute you step through the door.

All this event requires is a toned-down version of the Foxy Five. If you tend to go heavier on lipstick, try a soft berry pink with a neutral lip liner. If you just can't give up eyeliner, give the thick black pencil the night off and go a little lighter by dipping an extra-fine eye brush in gray shadow and gently dabbing it underneath your bottom lashes. The look is a bit more dramatic but still refined.

Foxy Overtime: If you want to quickly polish your nails, nothing says "I'm a keeper" more than a sheer, pale pink, or beige.

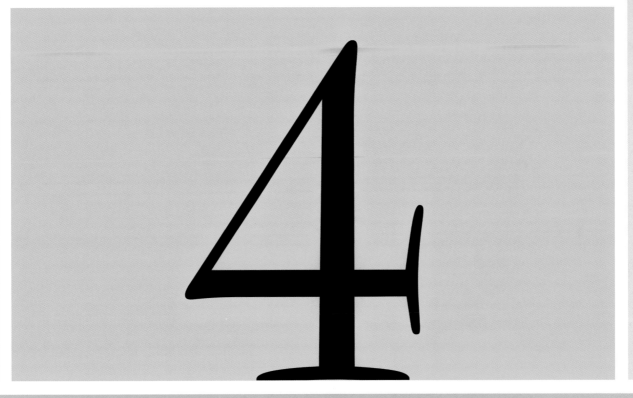

Foxy Free Time

Frumpy to Foxy: Weekend

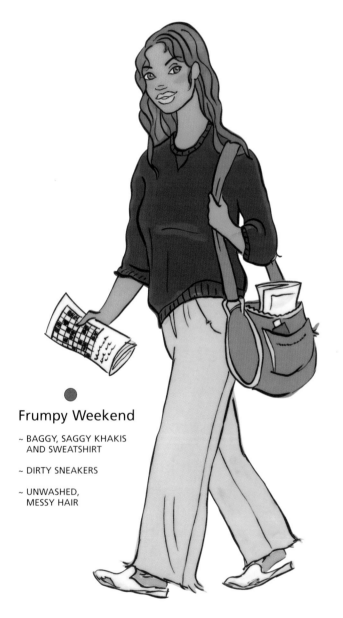

Frumpy Weekend

~ BAGGY, SAGGY KHAKIS
  AND SWEATSHIRT

~ DIRTY SNEAKERS

~ UNWASHED,
  MESSY HAIR

~Frumpy Fashion~

Ahhh, the weekend—at last! We can kick back, let loose, and wear whatever sloppy, pit-stained potato sack we want, right? Mmm, think again, foxettes. Those baggy khakis with the hole in the knee and the frayed hems don't quite give us the "lived-in preppy" look we had hoped for. Instead, they look like the pants we wear for house cleaning and other down-and-dirty tasks. Same for that saggy sweatshirt and the muddy sneakers with holes in them.

It's so easy to wake up late on a Saturday morning and pull on those XL knee-length gym shorts and that stained T-shirt you left crumpled on the floor last night. You just rolled out of bed, and unfortunately, you're going to look like it! You may just be going down to the corner to get a cup of coffee and a paper, but you don't want to look like you shuffled there in your sleep duds.

That stained canvas boat bag that you're using to haul crosswords, magazines, sunglasses, suntan lotion, and other goodies to and fro has got to go. Even if you're out and about on the weekends, running around like a lunatic, you can at least look like a foxy lunatic.

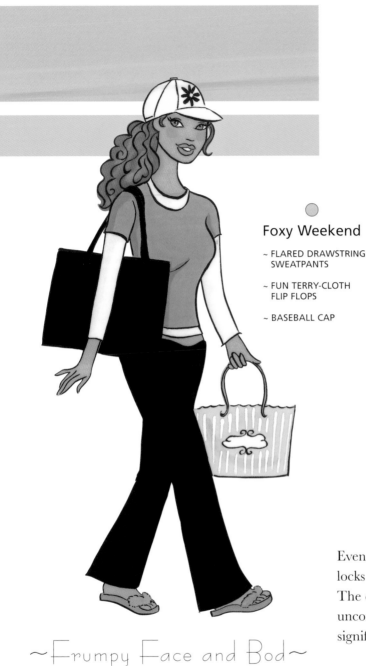

Foxy Weekend

~ FLARED DRAWSTRING
  SWEATPANTS

~ FUN TERRY-CLOTH
  FLIP FLOPS

~ BASEBALL CAP

~Frumpy Face and Bod~

Weekends are glorious because we get a break from our usual routine—that's what we love. But that doesn't mean foxettes can get away with doing nothing. The number one frump trap on weekends is uncombed hair. You don't have to wash it, you don't have to style it, but gals, you have to comb it!

Even those with super-short cuts should give their locks a once-over before facing the outside world. The only ones who should really see you in your uncombed state are your loved ones—pets and significant others—since they love you anyway.

As for that foxy face, sure you can squeeze by with minimal effort, but it does require a little. Whether your Sunday schedule is a good long workout at the gym, brunch with friends, or a matinee with the kids, avoid showing up with dark circles, blotchy skin, and pale, dry lips. Frumpiness never takes a holiday (or a weekend) off.

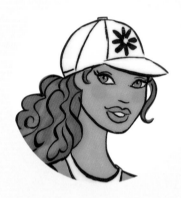

~Foxy Fashion~

Put some wow in your weekend, Foxy! The two foxy hall of fame choices for the weekend are jeans and sweats. Unless we've got a major to-do, we can't even think beyond those staples. Both allow you to be comfortable and casual, while still looking foxy and fabulous!

Our weekend jeans are different from our Friday work jeans or our going out jeans. Weekend jeans are the favorite, slightly faded, ultra-comfy, lived-in pair—the ones we'll wear until they've got holes in them and we can't wear them anymore. They're fitted, of course, but not too tight. After all, we have to allow room for the eggs benedict and extra caffe latte to settle in. Flared leg and boot-cut are both flattering styles, but go for what looks and feels best on you.

Another favorite is drawstring-waist sweatpants with a flared leg. Depending on your body shape and comfort level, slip into a slightly low waist, but stay away from a style that's too belly-baring. In the summer, look for a pair of capris. A "sweat skirt" is also a smart option for weekend-wear; choose one that's knee-length and super-comfy with a drawstring or elastic waist. Especially in hotter weather, this is a flawless foxy pick, and it works on most any body shape.

Pair any of the above with colorful cotton short- or long-sleeve layered tees—the number one favorite foxy weekend top. They're effortless and carefree. Experiment with funky color combinations; the weekend is the time to do it. Purple and pale pink, green and fuchsia, orange and blue. If it's chilly, throw on a cotton cardigan with a zip front. Give your feet a rest from the heels: Pamper them in rubber or terry flip-flops, cool retro sneakers, or espadrilles, and walk into a wonderful weekend.

In cooler weather, pair jeans with a casual wool turtleneck that hits at the hip and sneakers or comfortable low-heel ankle boots. If you need an extra layer, a hoodie or fitted twill jacket is the perfect way to round out your foxy weekend look. Add a soft cashmere scarf which feels luscious and luxurious and can also help warm you up.

A soft leather or canvas shoulder bag with short straps is ideal for running errands or brunching. You don't need anything too huge on the weekend, so give the mega-tote a few days off.

~Foxy Hair~

Shampooing every day can dry hair out, so give it a couple of days off. It will not only save you time, but it will save your shine. Rinse with a refreshing blast of cool water, then spritz your damp hair with leave-in conditioner. Your locks deserve a weekend, too, so give the blow-dryer a rest.

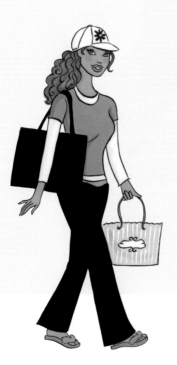

A foxette's favorite weekend accessory is a hat, which adds a foxy kick to your look and protects your skin from the sun. You'll never strike out in a baseball cap. If you have short hair, try a round hat with a short brim; for long hair, try a floppy straw hat.

~Foxy Face and Bod~

These are your two days off, so grooming should be as effortless as possible. The key? Next to nothing. Use only what you need to achieve a fresh-looking foxy face.

Pat cover-up on any blotchies and underneath your eyes, a little gel blush on each cheek, and tinted lip balm to moisturize those smackers. Cherry-flavored Chapstick has a subtle hint of color, and your lips will love any of the tinted balms by Kiehl's.

Frumpy to Foxy: Fitness

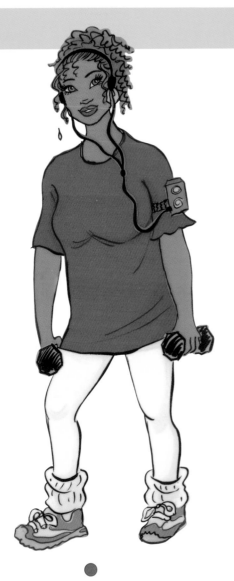

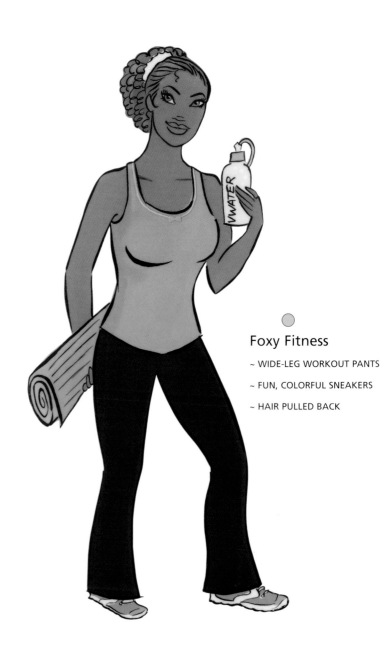

Frumpy Fitness

~ OLD, STRETCHED OUT T-SHIRT

~ UNFLATTERING LEGGINGS

~ LOOSE, MESSY HAIR

Foxy Fitness

~ WIDE-LEG WORKOUT PANTS

~ FUN, COLORFUL SNEAKERS

~ HAIR PULLED BACK

~Frumpy Fashion~

Let's face it, fellow foxettes, we've all got a little extra somethin' on our bods, but the answer is not to hide it underneath grim, gray sweatpants and a tent-sized Rolling Stones T-shirt. We may be going to the gym to sweat and suffer, but whether we're ninety pounds or 190, we can still look foxy while we're working out.

So toss the stretched-out, sweat-stained T-shirt and the saggy, baggy pants. You know, the ones that make our tush look like it ran for the hills. Same for those balloonlike, thigh-enlarging sweats with the tight elastic bottoms that leave red circles around your ankles. And white may be the ideal color for a wedding, but it's not the best choice for a workout. Those form-fitting white leggings show off every beloved roll, dimple, and floral panty line.

Another frump trap: biker shorts that look like they've sucked every ounce of air from your lungs. Even those fortunate few who can sort of pull it off don't look too comfortable.

And foxettes won't win any barbell beauty contests by pumping iron in those midriff athletic tops that display what we lovingly call our "chub-chub." We can't kid ourselves—they're more like bras than tanks, and they look best when covered up with a T-shirt (ditto for our chub-chub).

Those old, beaten-up, dirt-ridden sneakers with the frayed laces aren't only frumpy, but they're also probably so worn out that your tired feet will suffer even more after thirty minutes on the Stairmaster. And thick, oversized, clumpy socks could do double damage. For the sake of your hard-working feet, chuck 'em!

~Frumpy Face and Bod~

When we work out, we may have visions of looking like those incredible slow-motion athletes in the TV commercials—our hair whipping sexily to and fro—but after a little trial-and-error, we can chalk those images up to special effects. In reality, long, loose, damp hair just sticks to your sweaty face and gets caught in your mouth. There's got to be a better way to "just do it."

And how about caked-on makeup and drippy mascara, just for a visit to the gym? Foundation, lipstick, mascara, eye shadow, blush, the works! You're there to work out, not make out, so leave

Frumpy to Foxy in 15 Minutes

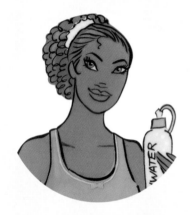

~Foxy Fashion~

Ready, set, foxy! 7:00 P.M. rolls around, and the last thing we want to do is hit the treadmill for forty-five minutes. The thought of getting our butts to the gym can be painful; fortunately, dressing for it couldn't be easier.

The greatest invention since chocolate chip cookie dough ice cream is wide-leg, stretchy cotton workout pants. They're flattering instead of

"fattering" on all shapes. And incredibly comfy, too.

Dark, solid colors like navy, charcoal, and black are more forgiving than light ones, and the flared bottoms somehow make us look a little longer and leaner. We also love the roll-over waistline that some of them have; it hides the extra pooch our stomachs acquired over the winter months. The best news is that these pants can take you right from the gym to lunch with the girls. You may just want to throw on a fresh T-shirt, or cover up with a hoodie, before hitting the road.

For those who like a little extra coverage or want to hide that dimpling that seems to catch up with us, slide into a pair of modern sweats. Instead of the balloon styles, opt for the kind with the elastic drawstring waist and

wide-bottom legs. The brilliant designer who decided to do away with those nasty elastic ankles is one smart cookie. You'll feel so foxy you'll wonder why you didn't think of them first.

Sport the bottoms with a tank top long enough to fully cover your midsection and even your hips, or try a cozy tee (not too tight and not roomy enough to take a swim in). If you're planning on doing some heavy cardio, you can wear that tiny, midriff workout top underneath for extra support.

Don't forget a really sturdy, "no bounce allowed" athletic bra, no matter what size you are. This means a bra that truly covers your breasts without any overhang creeping out on the sides. Otherwise, "the droopies" could the spackle and sparkle behind. That mountain of makeup isn't going to help you run that extra mile on the treadmill—more likely it'll run all over your face.

Bottom line: Don't turn your weekly gym outings into a fitness foul. Nothing is worse than dashing to the locker room and bumping into someone you know looking like a "frumpaholic."

catch up to you sooner than you'd like! Team a high-performance bra with the right bottoms; rid yourself of panty lines by sticking with thong undies.

For foxy feet, athletic shoes with cushioned soles will work for everything from jogging to jumping jacks (get them a half-size larger than normal since our feet swell when we sweat). Choose shoes in racy hues like red, orange, lime, or silver to spice up the look; staring down at our colorful sneaks while cycling uphill or on the treadmill can be a nice little pick-me-up.

Clean, thin, breathable socks or peds are much nicer to your toes than those awful extra-thick ones that leave your soles soaked in a puddle of sweat. Trust us, your feet with thank you. Who knew fitness could be so foxy!

~Foxy Hair~

A quick sweep of those tresses into a ponytail will keep your face from becoming a magnet for sticky hair. Or wrap your hair into a loose bun using a scrunchie or snag-free elastic, which won't tangle or tear your hair.

Short-haired foxettes cut their time down even more since they don't have to lift a finger; if anything, there's always a wide cotton headband.

~Foxy Face and Bod~

Some of us aren't overly fond of hitting the gym completely bare faced, even though fifteen minutes of working out is like your very own cosmetics bag, giving you rosy cheeks and all. You can choose to

go au naturel and let a few sexy (yes, sexy) beads of sweat give you a gorgeous glow.

Then again, it doesn't hurt to give yourself that "it doesn't look like I'm wearing any makeup, but I am" look by donning a touch of cover-up and waterproof mascara.

If you have the ability to turn into a human hose and look like you could water a lawn with all of that sweat, don't forget to always have along a trusty towel. Dab that drench, Foxy!

Wrap it up with a few swipes of deodorant and even a drop of light, freshly scented fragrance and go, Foxy, go!

Frumpy to Foxy: Lounging

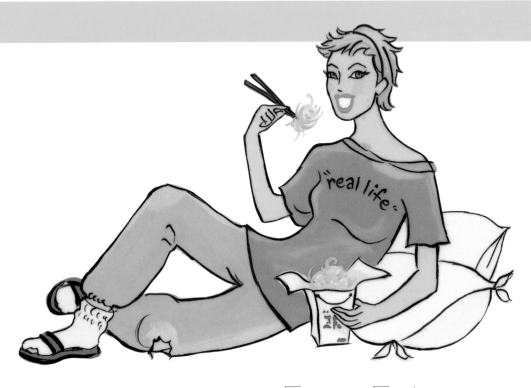

Frumpy Lounging

- ~ TOO-BIG TEE
- ~ BULKY SOCKS WITH SANDALS
- ~ MATTED, MESSY HAIR

~Frumpy Fashion~

It's time to kick off those shoes, slip into something soft and cozy, plop down on that mushy sofa, and forget about your nerve-grating, anal-retentive boss who was micro-managing you all day long—or tune out the kids who have been bouncing off the walls and driving you up the wall.

Even so, there's really no need for that bleach-stained, three times too big, shapeless T-shirt and the sweats with two large moth holes in the crotch.

Especially when lounging foxy style is such a cinch! And, maybe it's time to toss those dingy old slippers

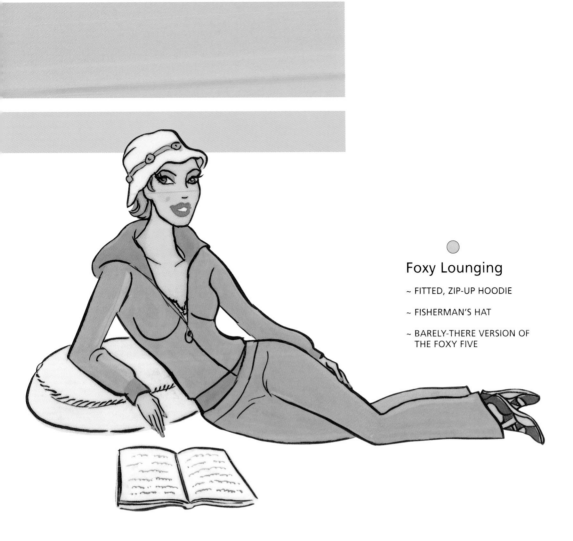

Foxy Lounging

~ FITTED, ZIP-UP HOODIE

~ FISHERMAN'S HAT

~ BARELY-THERE VERSION OF
  THE FOXY FIVE

that look like they've spent the better part of the day in the dog's mouth.

Maybe you and your best bud are planning a casual afternoon of at-home manicures and whipping up a batch of double fudge brownies. Or you and your guy are going to order some Kung Pao chicken and veggie fried rice, snuggle up, and watch a movie at home. That doesn't mean you have to lounge around in unbecoming jumbo jeans and a blousy T-shirt with wide, wing-like sleeves. Even worse, when you try to tuck it in, that bunchy bulk makes you look like you put on a few extras pounds. Tattered

plastic slides worn with thick athletic socks are another offender. Sure, you're just hanging at home, but it's quick and easy to do it with a touch of foxiness, so why not?

~Frumpy Face and Bod~

You may be struggling with allergies, recovering from a long day that has your eyes looking bloodshot and bleary, or simply feeling lazy, but just because you're relaxing and enjoying precious time off is no reason to miss out on a little foxiness. Besides, as

Mom always used to say, "You never know who you're going to run into, so always look your best." As usual, she was right.

There's got to be something we can do about greasy, two-day-old hair that's sticking up in back because we were too lazy to comb it out. As much as we try to kid ourselves, there's a big difference between sexily mussed hair and just plain matted, messy hair.

Lounging over the morning paper and a cup of herbal tea is a luxury, but if you were tossing and turning a lot the night before and have a little extra "sleep sweat" still stuck on you, don't just let it stay there. A quick rinse can turn frumpy to foxy, even if you and your family are the only ones around.

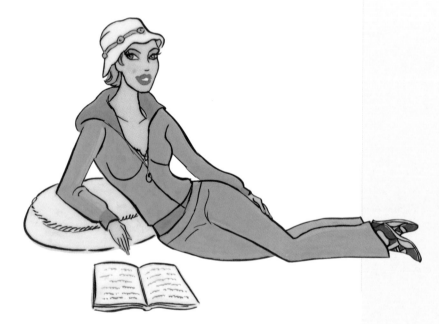

~Foxy Fashion~

Time to chill, Foxy! We love rare and precious "down time" and can't resist feeling foxy while we're kicking back and catching up on life. It's definitely possible to kick back and be comfortable while still maintaining your foxiness!

Even if you're enjoying some alone time while sprawled out on the living room floor flipping through magazines, there's something irresistible about doing it in boyfriend-style pajama bottoms and a spaghetti-strap tank—it's casual and loose, yet still sassy. Sure, no one's around to give you the once-over, but if they were, you'd bowl them over with your foxiness. A pair of fun, fuzzy slippers in bright pink or yellow will take you from the living room to the kitchen for bowls of popcorn in style.

A dash to the coffee shop to meet friends on a lazy Sunday afternoon certainly deserves a little foxing up. Feeling like a slug isn't enough to stop us from slipping into some wide-leg cotton pants with a drawstring waist and a zip-up hoodie shirt. It's such an easy, modern look—no wonder it's the foxette's most cherished weekend attire. Grab a small tote in a fun color to store all your essentials. Pair this outfit with colorful rubber flip-flops and an over-sized pair of sunglasses in a round or square shape and you'll be feeling it. Suddenly life's a little less sluggish and a lot more stylish!

There's a lot to love about running around in your favorite faded jeans and a worn-in cotton T-shirt that's been tossed around the dryer with fabric softener about fifty times. Look for tees that are a bit fitted—but not too tight. Add Velcro sneakers and you are the ultimate foxy lounge lizard! Everyone will be amazed at how comfortable and foxy you look!

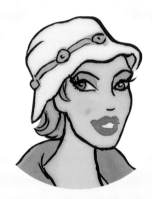

When the temperatures drop, chunky crew neck sweaters and velour sweatpants come to the rescue. All that's missing is a roaring fire and some hot cider. Even when you're chilling, you can look hot!

~Foxy Hair~

No matter what shape your hair is in—frizzies, greasies, and all—you can't go wrong with a trusty fisherman-style hat. This is especially true when you're just not in the mood to wash your hair, or during those times when it simply

decides to take on a mind of its own. A neat, high ponytail also gets the job done.

Versatile hair clips work wonders, too, for long or medium locks. Just twist your tresses and clamp them back for a tousled and totally irresistible look.

~Foxy Face and Bod~

Who's to say that lounging can't still be lovely? We know better . . .

The beauty of loungy days is that you can get away with a makeup-less face, especially when wearing a hat. Talk about saving time! If not, there's always a minimized version of the Foxy Five: a quick touch of cover-up, blush, and a swab of lip balm.

Frumpy to Foxy: Bedtime

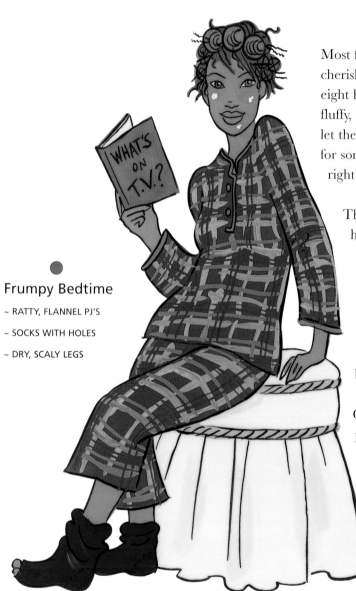

Frumpy Bedtime

~ RATTY, FLANNEL PJ'S

~ SOCKS WITH HOLES

~ DRY, SCALY LEGS

~Frumpy Fashion~

Most foxettes consider bedtime one of the most cherished times of day. Who doesn't appreciate six to eight hours of "me" time nuzzled beneath a big, fluffy, cloudlike comforter? So why do so many of us let the all-out frumps take over before we hit the sack for some good ol' shut-eye? Nighttime is not the right time to skip out on foxification.

Those old, ratty, plaid flannel pj's with the frayed hems and ripped pockets are buttery soft, but isn't it time to trade them in for something just a bit more alluring? And how some people can climb into bed wearing a stiff, starchy T-shirt remains a mystery. It may as well be one of those dreaded paper gowns from the doctor's office—convenient, maybe, but cozy, no way!

Of course, when a significant other is part of the picture, we don't go anywhere near our grandma-style undies. Yes, we own them; yes, they're extremely comfy; and yes, they serve several purposes (say, during that certain time of the month), but when he's lying next to his foxy girl, they're best tucked away, safely in the back corner of the underwear drawer, next to the workout bras.

Foxy Bedtime

~ SEXY NIGHTIE

~ SOFT, SILKY SKIN

~ HAIR PULLED BACK

Thick socks never seem very foxy, but during those nippy winter months they do come in handy. Just retire the tattered and holey ones that leave your toes popping. Softly swaddled feet will help you nod off into a night of sweet dreams.

~Frumpy Face and Bod~

It's so easy to ignore bedtime beauty rituals, especially when we're so pooped it's hard to even think about brushing our teeth. Much less a good, thorough flossing. Sounds like torture!

But remember, it'll only take a few minutes, and going to bed with bad garlic breath or dry, scaly, itchy legs is anything but foxy. Talk about an unrestful night's sleep. It's tempting to want to blast those breakouts with little dots of pasty drying lotion, but for the sake of foxiness, not when he's sleeping over. Save the chicken pox look for a night spent alone.

Unless, of course, he's a permanent keeper; in that case, maybe it's best to switch to a clear potion, or at the very least, keep those "pox" dots to a minimum.

The grandest of frumps? Jumping into bed with a face full of makeup. Who wants to wake up to eye shadow stains on the pillow and, even worse, clogged pores? You'll just end up working extra long and hard in the morning.

Frumpy to Foxy in 15 Minutes ⏱

~Foxy Fashion~

Nighty-night, Foxy! Aaaah, sleepy time . . . the perfect opportunity to fill up on zzz's and, of course, douse ourselves in all-out foxiness. And if a certain special someone is in the picture, there are no excuses not to crank things up every now and then.

Something's to be said about hopping into the sack with clean, silky, smooth skin and a dainty cotton chemise nightie in white, pale pink, light blue, or playful prints like polka dots. These nighties are sweet with just a touch of

naughtiness. And when you're tossing and turning, they won't get trapped between your legs the way full-length gowns do.

So what if you're dreaming solo? Nights are that much cozier when you slip into scrumptious skivvies. We're fond of fuller tushy coverage while at rest—like high-cut hipsters—since the skimpier styles can wake you up to a wedgie.

For a more casual feel, foxettes love a slightly fitted tank with boy-cut undies or loose pajama bottoms. Try borrowing your significant other's . . . ultra foxy.

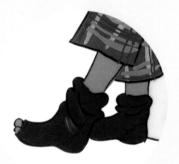

Feeling a bit randy? When you're in the mood to really turn things out, those demure, little sexy somethin's are a slam dunk. Channel one of the screen goddesses from the '50s and go for a sultry silk-and-lace teddy. They can be surprisingly comfy. And those stretchy mesh fabric tanks with matching panties in black, leopard, red, or hot pink will always punch it up.

Who knows, you may look so foxy, you won't get much sleep!

~Foxy Hair~

If you have medium or long hair that you don't wash every day, wrapping it up in a bun with a trusty scrunchie helps keep it from shooting off every which way while you sleep, and gives it extra body. What a time-saver the next morning: Just let your hair down, comb it out, and run some smoothing serum through your locks. A thirty-second blast of the blow-dryer will finish off the job. Bear in mind, no shampoo was required. Insert smile here.

~Foxy Face and Bod~

There's a reason they call it "beauty sleep." Hitting the hay doesn't require a long-winded routine of primp and prep, but a few quick tricks can leave you looking dreamy in the morning.

Getting ready to hit the sack can actually be a treat. First, a quickie shower, or, as we call it, "a rinser." Who wants to take the day's sweat and dirt to bed? We all get grimy, even if we're just plugging away at a computer all afternoon. A quick rinse takes just two minutes and gets us right into relaxation mode.

We know shaving can be a chore, but snuggling up between the sheets with several days of harsh stubble on your legs will leave your main squeeze suffering from razor burn. So spare thirty seconds to shave before you snooze.

Foxettes love to smother themselves in heavenly scented lotions and potions like Lubriderm or Johnson's Baby Oil Gel, the best defense for dry skin. If your feet are scaly and full of cracks, pile on the Vaseline, sleep in a pair of socks, and poof, like magic, wake up with tantalizing tootsies.

You may be asleep, but your facial cream isn't, so don't forget the moisturizer, and a hint of eye cream to stick it to those laugh lines. Follow up with inconspicuous blemish zapper, if needed, and a touch of lip balm (kept on the bedside table for easy access). Here's hoping for one gorgeous glow in the morning!

Frumpy to Foxy: Summer

~Frumpy Fashion~

Summertime, and the livin' is easy . . . or maybe not so easy if you don't have the right wardrobe to get you through those lazy, hazy days.

Who wears short shorts? Hopefully not you, Foxy. Well, at least not that short. If admirers can't tell whether you're wearing shorts or bikini bottoms, then those things are too itsy bitsy. They should flatter our beautiful backsides, not paint them.

Many of us have lived through long, hot summers in denim cutoffs, but pair them with a skimpy bikini top and you might be pushing it. Few gals can afford to walk around with their midriffs fully exposed, no matter how tan and tight they may be. When you stroll around town in this little getup, you might just end up looking like you "accidentally" lost your shirt. Oops.

Oversized pleated Bermuda shorts with cuffed bottoms can be just as frumpy. You'll look more like you're on our way to dig in the garden than splash down at an afternoon pool party.

We love tank tops, but make sure they fit snugly, especially around the arms. Let's hope they aren't gaping and giving the world a glimpse of the saggy beige bra you're sporting.

Sundresses are another summer must-have, but you're better off with one that won't have your breasts surfing freestyle. That flimsy fabric may be cool and breezy, but not without the right coverage. Sandals are the essential accessory, but not the heavy leather ones that make your feet look like prisoners.

And never sport socks with sandals; covering up those tempting tootsies defeats the purpose of wearing sandals in the first place. Shoes should be light, comfy, and carefree. After all, that's what summer is all about!

~Frumpy Face and Bod~

Summer is a time to let your hair down, but leaving it down might not be the best idea; sticky sweat will make it cling to your neck, face, and back.

Frumpy Summer

~ OVERSIZED BERMUDA SHORTS

~ HEAVY, CHUNKY SANDALS

~ BRA STRAPS SHOWING

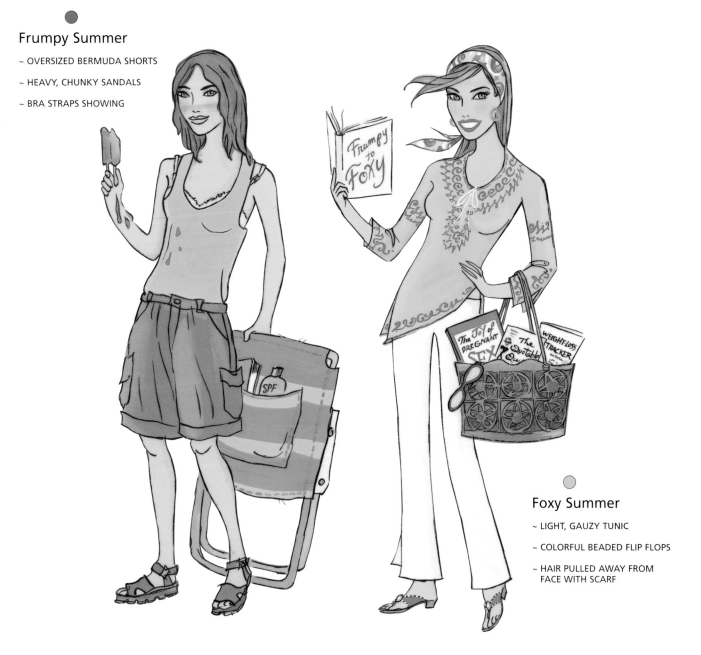

Foxy Summer

~ LIGHT, GAUZY TUNIC

~ COLORFUL BEADED FLIP FLOPS

~ HAIR PULLED AWAY FROM FACE WITH SCARF

Sweat also works hand in hand with its evil ally, heat rash, which pops up in the form of small red bumps or nasty breakouts. Not very foxy, especially in some tricky places, such as our arms and back. The thought of slipping into a swimsuit just got worse.

Some like it hot, but our swollen feet wouldn't agree. Watch out for stray corns, dry heels, or blistered toes.

Not to mention chipped or sloppy toenail polish. You can don the foxiest footwear in the world, but if your feet aren't foxy, what's the point?

Summer lips were made for sipping fresh lemonade and snacking on ice cream cones, so don't load them down with layers of heavy lipstick. The real scoop for summer is . . . lighten up!

~Foxy Fashion~

Now we're talking *hot,* Foxy! Swing into summer with a stash of mid-thigh linen or cotton shorts—flat front with some flare in the leg. If you have a mix of melon, powder blue, white, khaki, and black, you're good to go. Throw them on with a fitted linen or cotton tank, or a hip-length cap-sleeve tee, which gives sexy shape to the upper arms. A bright white top pops against any colored bottom. And be sure to invest in a good racerback or clear strap bra, so you can wear those tiny tanks with confidence.

If shorts aren't your style, or you're feeling a bit uneasy about your pasty thighs, opt for an above-the-knee denim skirt with a cotton camisole and hip-length, button-down shirt worn loose and open. Nothing could be easier than tossing on a delicate halter-neck sundress with flip-flops. The halter flatters your shapely shoulders and draws attention away from your arms and up to your face. Look for small patterns or textures; minimal prints minimize your bod. Some foxettes can go braless, but if you're a bit top-heavy, go with a strapless or convertible style.

Flat-front white pants will take you from Memorial Day through Labor Day and on. Look for crisp cotton chinos, full length with a slight flare. Pair them with a gauzy keyhole blouse or colorful silk tunic. Look for print or solid tops in classic summery colors like pinks, sage greens, and dusty light blues. Black and white is another hot color combo that will keep you looking cool.

A few colorful pairs of rubber and beaded flip-flops, wooden heel mules, ankle-strap espadrilles, and white sneakers are all the footwear you'll need. Summer bags are just as easy; go a bit more casual and playful than usual. We love a medium straw tote or short-handled canvas bag that slips over the shoulder. This is the season to travel light.

The same goes for jewelry: Less is more. Accessorize with a thick wood bangle, a trio of thin silver bangles to show off your tan, or a pair of small dangly earrings. To funk it up, play around with chunky turquoise or coral rings.

Finally, a foxette mustn't forget a good hat and favorite shades to shield her from the sun's searing rays. A straw or fisherman's hat with a medium brim goes with just about everything in your summer wardrobe. Even if you think you're not a hat person, use your head, Foxy—find a style that suits your personality and looks H-O-T!

~Foxy Hair~

As the mercury rises, hair should be ultra low-maintenance; spending too much time under the blow-dryer might make you melt. For medium or long locks, stay cool by keeping your hair away from your face and neck. Pull it into a back or side ponytail, or twist it into a large tortoise shell clip. Add some pizzazz with this quick trick using a colorful silk scarf: Roll it up into a flat three-inch-wide band and use it like a headband to keep hair slicked back and away from your foxy face.

Short-hair gals can go even shorter for summer. Smoothing pomade or hair gel will help keep your hair looking foxy instead of frizzy. A couple of tiny barrettes with butterflies will clip back bangs or stray hairs and add flavor to the season. Turn up the heat by rubbing shimmery hair wax onto chunks to give the illusion of highlights (so much quicker and cheaper than the salon!).

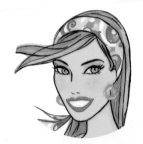

~Foxy Face and Bod~

Make sure those legs and underarms are silky smooth; even if you have to do it every day, a good shave is essential. Heat makes hair grow faster, so it takes a little extra TLC to stay prickly-free in the summer.

And since your skin can suffer a bit in the summer, use an acne-fighting body wash in the shower to prevent breakouts. Try a body lotion with a hint of shimmer which will give you a gorgeous glow.

Go light on makeup with a summer spin on the Foxy Five: tinted moisturizer with SPF, lightweight oil-free powder, shimmery pink blush or bronzer, waterproof mascara, and sheer lip glosses in pink, peach, or nude. The right powder is key to keeping you shine-free all summer. Loose powder applied with a big brush is best, since compacts can get cakey when mixed with moisture. Choose an ultra-sheer translucent powder with a silky texture, or if your face is flushed from the heat, try something with a slight yellow pigment to tone down the red. And replace your powder blush with a stick or liquid tint.

As for those foxy feet, treat them to weekly soaks in warm water spiked with baby oil. Then scrub them smooth with a pumice stone, and slather with cooling peppermint lotion. Punch up your pedicure with juicy warm-weather colors like coral, watermelon, or apricot. And we love French tips and sheer beiges for a clean look that mixes with any foxy outfit.

~Frumpy Fashion~

It's the much-anticipated night out with your fellow foxettes. You've been planning all week for this—your schedule is cleared (an almost impossible feat), reservations are made, a driver designated, and plans finalized to escape early from work. You'd think it would be practically impossible to frump out. Think again.

Girls' night out is to be honored, not disregarded. So don't bother slipping into the ordinary slacks and sweater ensemble you've worn to work all week—that spells boring boardroom, not bustling bar. While jeans can be quite foxy, wearing them with a T-shirt and flats makes a girl look like she's on her way to a baseball game, not a night of fruity cocktails and innocent flirting.

A shift dress is always a classic, but it's too conservative for an evening when you want to be a bit more daring and darling. A button-down cardigan sweater worn with a full-length skirt has many uses, but not for this evening of excitement.

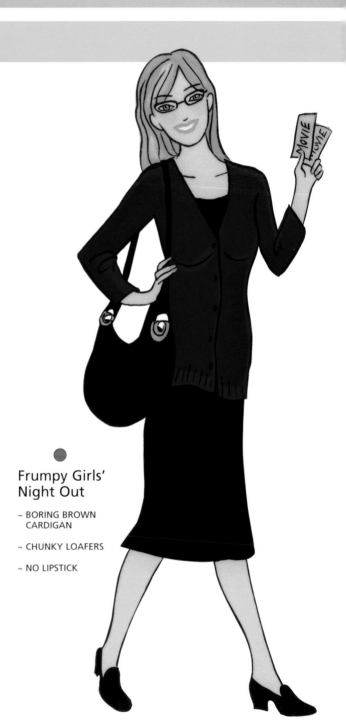

Frumpy Girls' Night Out

~ BORING BROWN CARDIGAN

~ CHUNKY LOAFERS

~ NO LIPSTICK

Night Out

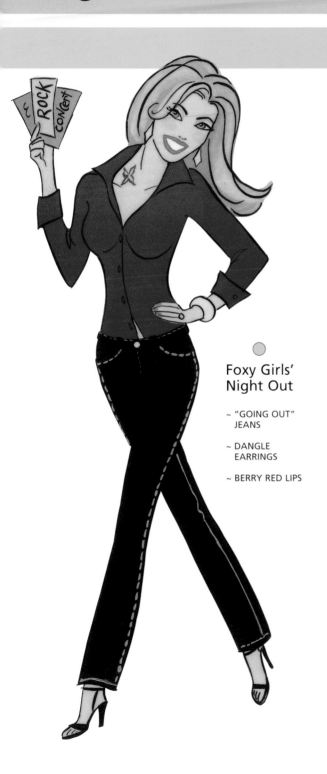

Foxy Girls' Night Out

~ "GOING OUT" JEANS

~ DANGLE EARRINGS

~ BERRY RED LIPS

Sneakers, however stylish they may be, won't add enough pizzazz to the night. Send 'em walking. Neither will chunky, clunky loafers, especially the ones with the two-inch-wide "Frankenstein" heel. There's no surer way to step out in frumpy style. Just as bad is the other extreme: Beware of vampy stilettos and mini skirts so skimpy your buns unexpectedly show up for the festivities. While it's nice to show off some cleavage and a little leg, you don't want to get too carried away and end up being mistaken for an exotic dancer.

Girls' night out is one of the most celebrated rituals of foxiness, so whether you're single or shacked up, give an evening out with your best buds all you've got.

~Foxy Face and Bod~

If there's an opportunity to go all out with hair and makeup, then hitting the town with the girls is it. But by Friday night, some of us are pretty pooped. It's easy to get stuck in the same old routine and

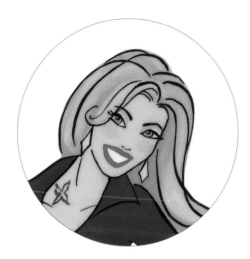

brush off a few minutes of dolling up. This isn't the time to do it.

One of the biggest offenders: no lipstick. It's a revved-up night out with the girls, after all, not a quick walk around the block with the dog. Chapstick doesn't really cut it, either. Save that for the surf or slopes.

Burning the midnight oil and missed a week's worth of shaving? Things could be getting pretty hairy. Remember, you're going for foxy, not furry. Your girlfriends will be the first to tell you that any foxette needs to nix the stubble if she wants to put her best foot forward.

Toward the end of the day, that perfume you spritzed on eight hours earlier has most likely taken on an interesting new scent, especially after mixing with the day's dirt and unavoidable office odors. Forgetting to freshen it up is a frumpy faux pas; you want to draw them in, not drive them away.

Frumpy to

~Foxy Fashion~

Paint the town red, Foxy! Go all out and make it a dazzling night. That slinky dress looks much better on you than curled up in the corner of your closet.

Kick things up several notches by breaking out that black, short to mid-length skirt with a slightly fitted, shoulder-baring top and fabulous open-toe, thin-strap stilettos.

In the mood to keep a bit more covered? Your favorite "going out" jeans never disappoint—the ones that lie just a bit lower on the hips with a straight leg. Finish off by sliding into a satiny or frilly blouse with detailing and, yes, those same "stop them in their tracks" stilettos, and you're good to go, Foxy. For foxettes who feel like they're going to stumble in stilettos, go as high as you can with an open-toe slide or ankle strap, and no more than a one-inch wide heel. When it comes to shoes, skinny = sexy.

Foxy in 15 Minutes ⏱

To really pump up the volume (on your breasts, that is), snap on a push-up or padded bra. Who doesn't appreciate a little lift?

Add a piece or two of the jewelry that's been collecting dust on your dresser. Now's the time to break out those colorful pieces you keep telling yourself you're going to wear but never do. Bangles, cuff bracelets, chokers, beaded necklaces, large rings, and long dagger-style earrings will add glam to your getup.

Feeling extra playful? Pile on a few more bangles. The sound of your bracelets will add a funky beat to the night . . . and your friends will always know where you are.

~Foxy Hair~

Give your hair a few extra spritzes of volumizer on the roots when you blow it dry in the morning. Right before you go out, refresh with a bit of light hair spray and a quick shot of the hair dryer. Then use your fingers to crunch and curl hair as you dry for a tousled and slightly wild look; this will work for any length hair. Finish with a shot of glossing spray all over.

~Foxy Face and Bod~

If you usually wear a colorless lip balm during the day, girls' night out gives you a reason to add some kick. That goes for all of your makeup, so try taking the Foxy Five up a notch or two.

Go a bit heavier on the blush and mascara. Whatever you do, deck those lashes out with at least two coats. Follow with a light brushing of shimmery brown or gray powdered shadow directly underneath and above your lashes, sticking close to the lash line. If your lips look anything but luscious, saturate them in a rich, creamy color like berry red or dark pink, or go for a mouth full of high-gloss nude shine. Make sure your lips are soft and velvety all night long.

If you have a few extra minutes, go into Foxy Overtime and decorate your nails with a quick coat of sexy, deep-colored polish such as dark plum or cherry red. It will transform your hands from dainty day to naughty night. For the same effect on the rest of your body, dust some shimmering body powder around your neck, shoulders, and chest.

Don't forget to freshen up your everyday fragrance, or switch to a slightly richer, evening scent for this foxy occasion.

One final touch takes you from babe to bombshell: Turn up the heat by sticking a crystal tattoo on the back of your shoulder or near your collarbone. Talk about a clever conversation starter!

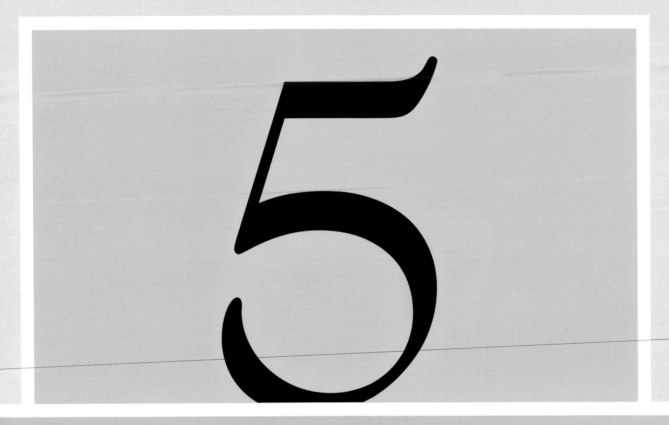

5

Foxy Festivities

Frumpy to Foxy: Cocktails

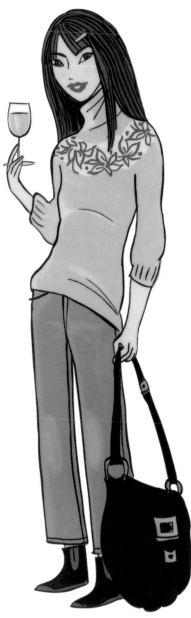

Frumpy Cocktails

~ FADED JEANS

~ FLAT ANKLE BOOTS

~ OVERSIZED BAG

~Frumpy Fashion~

Get the champagne flutes ready! You're having a cocktail party. The seared chicken sticks and crab cakes are ready to go, so why the blah outfit for such a festive evening?

A weary, white, workday shirt and khaki slacks worn with flats aren't going to mix with all that toasting and laughing. Same for that turtleneck with the snags you hope no one will notice, paired with faded jeans and boots. That outfit's okay if for running errands, but not for this foxy evening.

On the other hand, a summery pink and yellow sundress and floral sandal ensemble sets the mood for an afternoon picnic at the park, not a sophisticated evening of Burgundy and Brie. And that navy knee-length skirt with the matching boxy blazer? Finish it off with neutral-colored hose and square-toe shoes, and

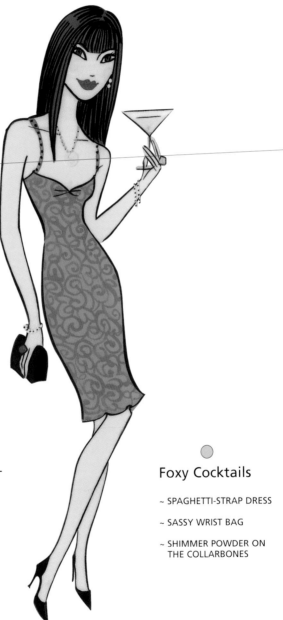

perhaps it would be better suited for a hearing on Capitol Hill than a cocktail party.

If the gathering is an artsier affair, you may be tempted to wear jeans with a crocheted halter top and platform shoes. But this funky getup won't get a foxette anywhere with the bohemian crowd that has assembled to sip, see, and be seen. It's a cocktail party, not a rock concert.

And, wouldn't you know it, you forgot to switch handbags, so you're still carrying the same tattered one you've been lugging around all day. In fact, the other half of the banana muffin from this morning is still inside, along with all those crumbs that have now attached themselves to your lipstick and wallet. Somehow crumbs and cocktails just don't mix. This is a cocktail party, not a business lunch. Get ready to shake up more than just a martini.

Foxy Cocktails

~ SPAGHETTI-STRAP DRESS

~ SASSY WRIST BAG

~ SHIMMER POWDER ON
  THE COLLARBONES

~Frumpy Face and Bod~

Even if you've been running errands since noon, the "haven't-combed-my-hair-all-day" look just doesn't fit with a cocktail party. And who knows what you may have picked up along the way: a few stray leaves mangled up in the back of your head after brushing past that oversized bush in the driveway, a smattering of sticky fruit juice left behind when Junior playfully tugged your locks during lunch? It's okay to be busy—even a bit frazzled—but you can never make an entrance at a cocktail party looking frumpy!

A set of colorless, chapped lips isn't the greatest accessory either. It'll look more like you spent the afternoon on the ski slopes whipping along at thirty miles per hour. Talk about needing to wet your whistle . . .

It's guaranteed that at any see-and-be-seen soiree you'll be hobnobbing with lots of friends, old and new. Nothing's frumpier than shaking hands with the hostess or fellow partygoers only to look down and notice that the rosy nail color painted on a week ago is half gone and those thick cuticles have inched their way up your nails. Uh oh. You immediately look down at your sandal-clad feet and suddenly they don't look so pretty, either. The pink polish has turned pasty orange, and now that it's started to peel away, those toenails look more like pieces of abstract art.

Frumpy to

~Foxy Fashion~

Cheers, Foxy! Schmooze the night away!

It's almost impossible to go wrong with a knee-length skirt in black, maroon, navy, or chocolaty brown (fitted or A-line flare, which flatters all body types). Throw on a soft, tailored long-sleeve round-neck sweater and ankle-tie heels. When you don't have time to rack your brain about what to wear, this enduring little ensemble will always be there right by your side, or rather, resting safely in your closet. It's classic and forever foxy.

When you want to really turn it out, try a tank or spaghetti-strap knee-length dress in a rich shade of magenta, dark sage green, dusty purple, periwinkle blue, or any other favorite color. You'll cause the guys in the room to spill their drinks! And these colors will pop in a sea of basic black.

Foxy in 15 Minutes ⏱

If, like many foxettes out there, you have a not-so-secret shoe fetish, slip into an open-toe mule with a two-inch-plus heel and let those pretty painted piggies shine! If the thought of showing off your feet leaves you less than footloose, then dainty ballet flats are a good bet.

The sparkling cherries on top? An oversized bauble ring worn all by itself makes a statement. It doesn't matter if the gem is real or fake, as long as it spells fun. Garnish your neck with a large flat circle pendant necklace—now we're talkin' foxy!

Before heading out the door, grab a small- to medium-sized shoulder or sequined wrist bag and fill it with the Foxy Few: keys, driver's license, lipstick for retouching, mini powder compact, mints, and a few dollar bills in case you need to tip the bartender.

~Foxy Hair~

If the day has taken a toll on your do, refresh by gently brushing with a soft natural bristle brush like those made by Mason Pearson, followed by scented hair spray.

Make yourself the toast of the town. Spare a little Foxy Overtime by blowing your shoulder-length or long hair out smooth and slick.

Foxettes with short hair can make sparkle the theme of the evening by adding a few twists of the curling iron for wavy accents, and using shimmery hair wax to add shine.

~Foxy Face and Bod~

Keep with the theme by brushing your lids with peach or beige shimmer shadow and dabbing your cheeks with a touch of highlighting cream in a very light pink or bronze. Finish off with a light dusting of shimmer powder along your collarbone and chest, and around the corners of your eyes. You'll have a rosy glow to match that cranberry Cosmo.

A creamy deep red or magenta lip color is irresistible. A few final foxy touches will make you look like one tall drink o' water: Give your legs a sexy shine with a quick coat of body oil or shimmering lotion, indulge in the foxy Five-Minute Manicure if needed, and spritz your bod with a shot of a mysterious fragrance like Narciso Rodriguez or Hanae Mori.

Bartender, make that a double!

Frumpy to Foxy: Dinner

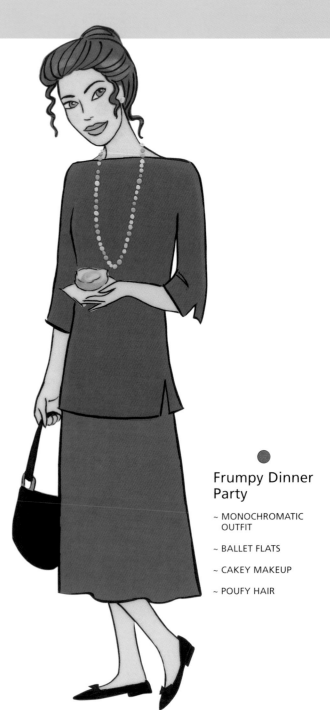

~Frumpy Fashion~

Dinner parties are endless fun, whether you're playing hostess or guest. But regardless of what's on the menu, make sure you don't show up looking frumpy, or you may not be invited to stay for cake and cappuccino.

A dinner party should feel special, even if it's something you do once a week. Stay away from jeans. Sure, you could dress them up, but someone put a lot of effort into the delicious dinner you're about to devour, so you should put in some effort as well.

It's also a good idea to avoid the monochromatic look. All one color from top to toes is bland and makes a girl look like an unimaginative dresser. Show up in a green skirt and matching green sweater, and you may look like a lizard. And an all-black turtleneck and slacks ensemble could be too somber for this intimate dining experience. You want to look like you're at a feast, not a funeral, so cook up a little something special and add the right dash of color to the mix.

Frumpy Dinner Party

~ MONOCHROMATIC OUTFIT

~ BALLET FLATS

~ CAKEY MAKEUP

~ POUFY HAIR

On the other hand, don't take the dress-up game too far: Frilly party dresses may work for a more extravagant affair, but in this kind of a cozy setting, you'll make the other guests feel uptight and underdressed.

When you're invited to a dinner party, be it large or small, you have to put a little foxy in your fashion. That way, you can ensure that they're roasting the chicken and not you!

~Frumpy Face and Bod~

Don't overdo the cakey makeup, or you'll look like you have more layers than the lasagna. Remember, people get "up close and personal" at dinner parties, so makeup shouldn't be maxed out.

Same for hair: You don't want to look like you have a cream puff on your head! Foxettes never look like they spent hours getting ready for a laid-back evening of wining and dining. No matter what the occasion, foxy style should always seem effortless.

Foxy Dinner Party

~ BLOUSE IN BRIGHT PUCCI-ESQUE PATTERN

~ LAYERED GOLD NECKLACES

~ STRAPPY SANDALS

~ BRONZY BROWN SHADOW FOR EYES

~Foxy Fashion~

You are one delicious-looking dish, Foxy!

What could be better than gathering with friends and family, gorging on gourmet goodies, drinking good wine, and talking the night away while R&B rhythms fill the room? Do things right, and you'll be twice as appetizing as the grilled salmon that's being served.

Make sure you're the main course of the evening, starting with taupe wide-leg pants with a cuffed leg. Look for wool, rayon, or gabardine in a lower-cut style that sits on your hips, rather than your waist, which looks more contemporary and sexier. The cuff adds elegance for the evening. Slide into a fitted silk button-down in a funky or graphic Pucci-esque pattern, and on your foxy feet, slip on 1940s-style T-strap heels. Adorn your ears with gold hoop earrings, and you're a feast for the eyes.

For a dressier dinner, look tasty in slim white gabardine pants, a sleeveless chiffon blouse in dusty blue or pearl gray, and silver leather strappy sandals. Complete the look with a beaded clutch, a chunky silver cuff bracelet, and silver dagger earrings. White is an unexpected night-time alternative to basic black, and the silver and gray accents will add sparkle.

During cooler seasons, trade that poufy party dress for a rich chocolate brown knee-length suede skirt with a cream, pale blue, or burgundy V-neck sweater and knee-high tan leather boots with killer heels—a smokin' look for any sumptuous soiree. Suede is sexy no matter how you wear it, and it's thick enough to forgive any rolls and ripples (love that!). Accessorize with a trio of layered gold necklaces of varying lengths,

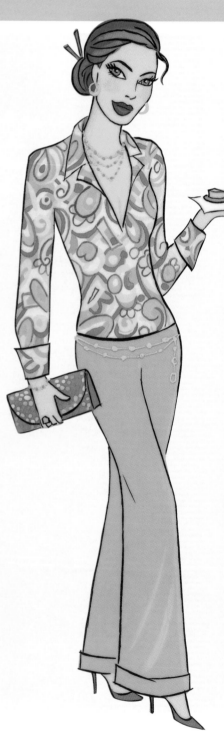

and a stack of thin gold rings on one finger. Take along an autumn-colored wrap—with burgundy, rose, cream, cognac, or soft gold shades—and a vintage-style hand-bag to add some attitude.

For those foxettes who are partial to that dinner party favorite, the little black dress, spice things up by ditching the standard sheath style for a more modern cut. Try an asymmetrical off-the-shoulder neckline . . . or don a drapey wrap dress with thin-heel Mary Janes and a chunky silver necklace to fill in that delicious décolletage. If you're feeling a little more daring, add some zest with a plunging down-to-there V-neck, dramatic bell sleeves, or a sexy side slit. Black doesn't have to be boring!

Finally, whether it's serve-yourself or sitdown, foxettes never show up at a dinner party empty-handed. Toast your host or hostess with a small gift that can be used to sweeten up the evening—a box of delicate chocolates or a bottle of your favorite after-dinner drink should get you invited back for seconds.

It's as easy as that to cook up a mouthwatering look in no time!

~Foxy Hair~

Don't overdo hair for a dinner party. In fact, don't do much to it at all. Dinner parties shouldn't be fussy affairs, so don't fuss.

Wrap long hair into a loose bun in back and hold it in place with chopstick-style hair pins. For med-ium hair, try a sexy asymmetrical style: Clip the top of one side back with a small barrette and let the other side hang loose. Slick short hair back using hair wax with a light tropical scent, and you won't even need perfume!

~Foxy Face and Bod~

The Foxy Five gives you the ideal base for any dinner party. If your skin is feeling a bit dry by the end of the day, spritz with a moisturiz-ing facial spray (key ingredient: aloe vera) before foxifying your face to prevent caking and flaking.

Try a smoky eye shadow to go with your free 'n easy yet foxy evening look. Brush a bronzy brown or pearl gray eye powder underneath your lashes. Balance it out with a sheer wine-colored gloss on your lips. Now who's smokin'!

Frumpy to Foxy: Holiday

~Frumpy Fashion~

Santa Claus is coming to town, Foxy, so break out the red, white, and green. Just be sure you're nice and not naughty . . .

We love any chance to wear red, one of our favorite foxy colors. But you have to be careful not to dress like one of Santa's elves. Red from head to toe is a no-go. Red and green plaid may be in keeping with the season's festive palette, but you need to be careful you don't come off looking like a lumberjack whose job is cutting down trees instead of decorating them.

The holidays are a time to get playful with fashion, but don't overdo the kitsch factor. A sweater with a huge fake fur collar and fluffy cuffs may leave you looking like Frosty the Snowman. And white patterned pantyhose with a dark dress can create a human "candy cane" look that's not too appetizing.

As for those oversized earrings shaped like Christmas trees that light up and play "O Tannenbaum," the kids may think they're cool, but in an adult crowd, they just look kooky. Overload on the jewelry, and you may resemble an evergreen suffering an overdose of tinsel.

The holiday should be merry and bright, so don't be a grinch! Go foxy, not frumpy, and your Christmas will be festive for sure.

~Frumpy Face and Bod~

It's December and you may be dreaming of a white Christmas, but that doesn't mean your skin should be pale as new fallen snow. Too little sunlight or too many holiday parties, can render that gorgeous complexion limp and lifeless. Too much makeup isn't very foxy, either.

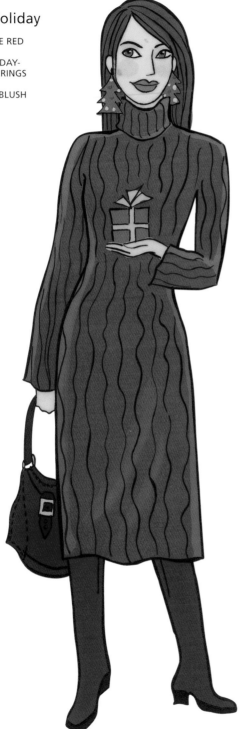

Frumpy Holiday

~ HEAD-TO-TOE RED

~ KOOKY HOLIDAY-
  THEMED EARRINGS

~ OVER-DONE BLUSH

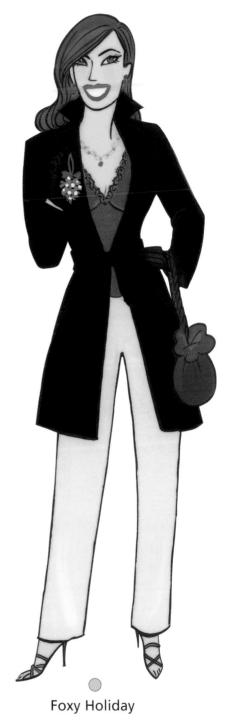

Foxy Holiday

~ IVORY WOOL PANTS

~ VELVET WRIST-BAG

~ SWEETHEART ROSE
  BEHIND ONE EAR

We love holly green clothing, but don't carry the color theme too far—like to your makeup. Before you put that green eye shadow on, remember that it's a hard look to pull off. Careful with those reds, too; you want to pick the shade of red lipstick or rouge that's right for your skin tone. And make sure not to overdo it on the red blush, or you'll resemble a Raggedy Ann doll with patches of cherry war paint on your cheeks.

Wintery weather can leave your skin dull and ashy.

Frumpy to Foxy in 5 Minutes

~Foxy Fashion~

Deck the halls, Foxy! We're making our list and checking it twice, and it will definitely include a sleighful of items in velvet and cashmere.

A pair of black boot-cut velvet pants is the place to start. Velvet is one of the foxiest fabrics on earth and instantly adds a festive sheen. Top it off with a long cashmere turtleneck in plum or teal (a cheery spin on basic red and green) or a cream satin blouse. Deck your feet in pointed-toe black leather boots or pumps for a dressy finish.

Another look we foxettes love is flowing ivory wool pants with a silk cranberry-colored blouse. Try out a wrap style to flatter your feminine form, or go with a gauzy bell-sleeve or keyhole blouse if you want a looser look. Gold or gunmetal metallic strappy dress sandals or suede camel pumps will coordinate with the merry palette and perfect this super-foxy outfit.

For slightly dressier holiday affairs, try a swingy black below-the-knee velvet skirt with a slim crewneck or cross-your-heart sweater in a rich jewel tone. Even if you love an all-black ensemble, the pop of color will wrap you up like a pretty package. Decorate your legs in sheer black hose or black fishnets and high-heel Mary Janes.

During the holidays, break out those Christmasy colors—wine and burgundy, forest green, silver and gold. If you feel like kicking it up a notch, try a deep fuchsia or lime green, a contemporary spin on red and green. Mix any of these with cream or black, and you've got a foolproof holiday formula.

Festive foxettes love velvet or raw silk bags for the holidays. Try a small drawstring wrist bag or a beaded clutch.

Add a few "ornaments" to your outfit with holiday jewelry. Teardrop earrings with peridot or rubies will add some twinkle to your yuletide without getting too into the spirit of the season. They're so much foxier than those long candy cane earrings!

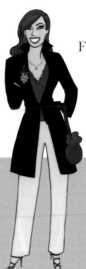

On the other hand, over-moisturizing can leave skin shining like a silver ball ornament. You don't want people to see you and start humming "if you ever saw it, you would even say it glows." Hey, Rudolph!

Finally, the holidays are a joyful time full of parties, but be careful all that holiday mulled wine doesn't stain your teeth red, or you'll be singing "all I want for Christmas is my two front teeth!"

Finally, we couldn't make it through the holiday season without a cool-weather coat and a few foxy winter accessories. The best defense in the cold weather is black; it holds up against snow storms, seasonal parties, and more. Find a three-quarter-length wool coat that's fitted at the waist and maybe even belted, like a slim Santa! Add a colorful wool or cashmere scarf around your neck; a dark pink or gentle melon tone will warm you up. And black leather gloves will keep your foxy fingers toasty.

Now that you're foxified, pour yourself a glass of eggnog and have yourself a merry little Christmas!

~Foxy Hair~

All we want for Christmas are foxy finishing touches—a small sequined red barrette, or a red sweetheart rose tucked behind one ear.

~Foxy Face and Bod~

'Tis the season, so use a richer moisturizer and creamier foundation to even out blotchy winter skin and provide extra protection from the cold, blustery weather. Dot eye cream around your eyes before applying cover-up so you don't end up looking like a frosted fruitcake.

Find a luminizing rosy blush to get you through the season (and those post-holiday January blahs). Dust a big round brush over the blush, shake off any excess, and stroke lightly over the apples of your cheeks. If you're afraid of going too heavy with a powder blush, blend a single dot of liquid color like Benetint from Benefit upward from the apple of your cheek for a natural freezing-weather "flush."

If you have any hopes of getting smooched under the mistletoe, your lips should be dolled up in rich red color. A moisturizing lipstick will chase away any chaps and flakes.

Frumpy to Foxy Formal:

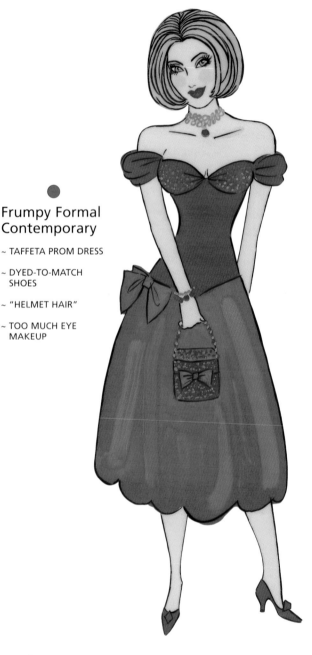

Frumpy Formal Contemporary

~ TAFFETA PROM DRESS

~ DYED-TO-MATCH SHOES

~ "HELMET HAIR"

~ TOO MUCH EYE MAKEUP

~Frumpy Fashion~

Any affair that's been dubbed black-tie makes you feel like Cinderella. But one false move, and the fairy tale can turn into a harsh, frumpy reality.

That "formal attire required" invite isn't an opportunity to dust the mothballs off that old prom dress that squeezes your breasts and hips into distorted lumps. And too much lace will make you look like a prom date from hell or like you belong perched on top of a wedding cake. Either way, not a good thing. All that glitters is not gold: Too much shiny fabric, too many sequins and cubic zirconia accents, and everyone at the bash will be blinded by something other than your beauty. If you want to impress Prince Charming, leave the tiara at home.

You might also need to face the fact that the single pair of trusty dress shoes you own may not be the right fit for this formal affair. A black heavy sandal doesn't go with a pale, delicate dress. Dyed-to-match shoes are just as bad; they have "bridesmaid" written all over them.

Bad pantyhose are the sour cherry on top of this festively frumpy sundae. They may seem like a necessity of female life, but they aren't, especially if

Contemporary

they're snaggy, saggy, and baggy. You'd be better off in your bare feet! Particularly if a certain someone shows up with that glass slipper . . .

~Frumpy Face and Bod~

We're pretty sure that invite didn't say "helmet hair optional"—and even if it did, opt out! Just say "I don't" to that stiff, formal do.

A more formal face may be appropriate for such a dressy evening, but formal makeup can be tricky, so better safe than sorry. A black-tie face doesn't mean looking like you have a black eye. That "smoky" shadow look pictured in your favorite fashion magazine looked foxy, but somehow when you tried to mimic it on your own fabulous face, it left you looking a little like Cat Woman.

And danger, foxettes: Beware of lipstick on the teeth, which is often an unfortunate side effect of glopping on too much lip goo.

Even though you intended to add just a little extra to your festive face, it's easy to get carried away and go too far for this swanky affair. There's a reason all those Tinseltown starlets trust professionals for those red carpet outings!

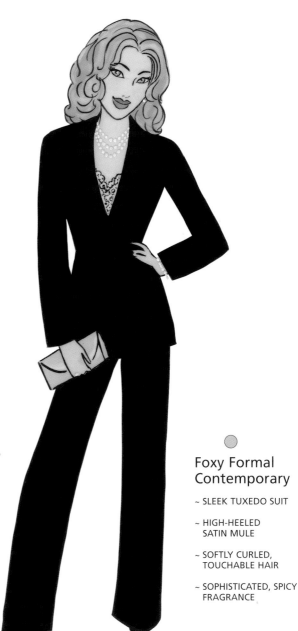

Foxy Formal Contemporary

~ SLEEK TUXEDO SUIT

~ HIGH-HEELED SATIN MULE

~ SOFTLY CURLED, TOUCHABLE HAIR

~ SOPHISTICATED, SPICY FRAGRANCE

Frumpy to Foxy in 15 Minutes

~Foxy Fashion~

Sweep them off their feet, Foxy! Be the belle of the ball.

A sleek tuxedo suit is the perfect contemporary spin on black tie—dressy but not froufrou. Underneath, tuck a light, lacy camisole (just a whisper of lace) or a silky tank with a little detail. Something in rich creamy tones works best because it doesn't overpower your look. Keep it clean: It's better to add a hint of color through accessories than through key clothing pieces.

Whether you're headed to a fancy fundraising dinner or a holiday bash, walk the red carpet in a strappy black sandal with a three-inch heel, or a high-heeled closed-toe satin mule. Either will be a foxy feminine finish to your luxe-tux look. This is the time to try a shoe with beaded or sequined embellishments; glittery accents look better on accessories than plastered all over your clothing. You don't need stockings, but if you can't resist, very sheer black hose work well.

Top off your glam getup with glitzy accents. Diamonds may be a girl's best friend, but when it comes to black tie, it's hard to go wrong with pearls. If you want to take the sex appeal up a notch, try layering long and short necklaces and combining pearls with silver or gold chains for a slightly opulent look. Pearl or diamond earrings—studs or long teardrops—are all you need to look like a bejeweled black-tie babe.

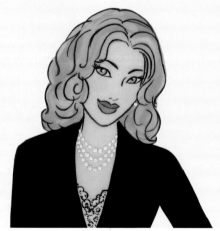

Finally, a satiny clutch serves as a slim, sexy carryall for your fancy foxified evening. This is the place to play with color, like magenta or gold.

Now, let's hope your date is as dashing as you are!

~Foxy Hair~

Black tie may be formal, but it can still be fun. Hair should be loose and feminine.

For those with longer hair, curl a few strands to give it a tousled look and pull it loosely into a wispy updo. This may require Foxy Overtime, if you have it.

For medium-length hair, leave it loose and use a jumbo-sized brush to give the ends a nice soft curl. Flip pieces in different directions, so you end with a soft tousled look and not a pageboy.

Foxettes with shorter hair can toss in a little gloss for shine. If you want to amp it up even more, adorn your do with a small rhinestone or pearl bobby pin.

Hair spray is key for black-tie evenings, since you want your locks to look polished. Choose a light spray with a slight sheen, such as Sebastian Shaper, so your hold will be soft and shiny, not hard and helmety.

~Foxy Face and Bod~

Fire up the Foxy Five with some stardust. Add shimmer for the evening to make yourself look—and feel—more festive than usual. A dusting of sparkly powder on your chest and collarbone and a touch on your eyes will give you just enough glow to go, whether you're sitting down to a six-course meal or boogying to big-band tunes all night long.

If you want to go with a smokier eye, use a thin, stubby brush dipped in deep plum eye shadow to accentuate your upper and lower lash line. Shadow is much easier to work with than waxy black eye liner.

Give your eyes an extra coat of volumizing mascara, and take the time to line your lips with wine-colored pencil to give them extra oomph. Experiment with wine or deep rose lipstick; choose one with a creamy texture so it won't end up caking onto your teeth.

Even if you're not a big perfume lover, a formal affair is the time to try out a scent. Go with something sophisticated, slightly spicy or musky.

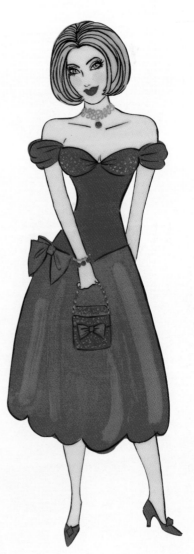

Frumpy to Foxy Formal:

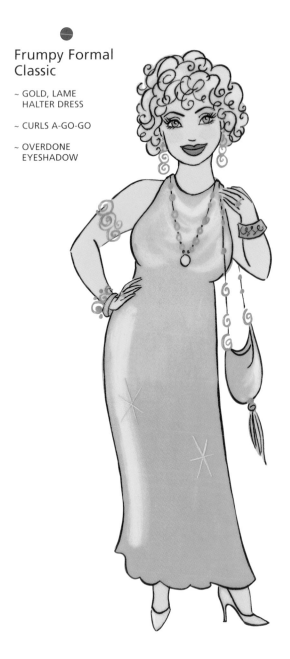

Frumpy Formal
Classic

~ GOLD, LAME
  HALTER DRESS

~ CURLS A-GO-GO

~ OVERDONE
  EYESHADOW

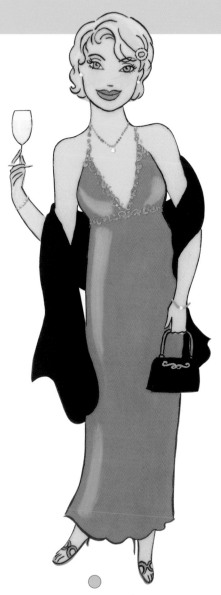

Foxy Formal
Classic

~ EMPIRE WAIST, A-LINE DRESS

~ DELICATE DIAMOND PENDANT
  AND STUD EARRINGS

~ VOLUMIZING MASCARA

Classic

~Frumpy Fashion~

As much as a foxette loves a good party, one of the problems with black-tie events is that unless you go to a lot of these things, you probably have a limited wardrobe for formal affairs. And since you don't want to spend hundreds of dollars for a dress you might wear one night a year, you're stuck in a frumpy bind.

That can sometimes lead to wearing the only "fancy dress" in your closet, even if it's a style that went out with blue leisure suits and hip huggers. That gold lamé halter dress was the must-have foxy frock for disco dancing in the 19'70s, but it's an antique today. The only women who can pull off that look are supermodels and the extremely fashion forward.

The long-sleeved busty beaded number with the pleated floor-length skirt might qualify as black tie, but "matronly" probably isn't the adjective you hope to inspire. One false move can take you from fashionable to old-fashioned.

You may be excited about a night fox-trotting to live jazz music, but watch out for your choice of dancing shoes. Patent leather heels are quirky in their own way, but they may have you frump-trotting instead.

As for accessories, black tie doesn't mean bejeweled from head to toe. Bracelets on both wrists, rings on every finger, and enough necklaces to fill a small bank vault aren't the most surefire way to formalize your look.

~Frumpy Face and Bod~

Warning, foxettes: Watch out for curls a-go-go! Pouf and elevation do not equate to foxiness when it comes to your hairstyle. There's no reason those lovely locks should look like they were tortured into submission.

And the last thing you want is to feel shellacked for this special evening. Too much of anything— hair spray, rouge, lipstick, or perfume—can leave you looking frumpy and fussy instead of foxy.

This isn't the night to try out tons of fake eyelashes or blue or green eye shadow to match your seafoam-colored frock. Unless you're a true pro, you could end up looking like a drag queen.

~Foxy Fashion~

Save the last dance for me, Foxy!

If you want to stun on this special evening, do it in a classic and flattering floor-length dress. Styles that work well on different body shapes are an empire waist with a gentle flare, a strapless A-line, or a spaghetti-strap dress with a deep V-neck. You may have to spend a small fortune, so make sure it's a style and color you can live with for more than a few years.

Candy-colored tones can look too trendy and seasonal, so stick with classics like black, red, neutral creams, and bronzy tones for sure-fire foxiness. And don't be dull: Look for a dress with a hint of interesting detail or unique styling along the neck or sleeves, so when you make your grand entrance, people will really notice. Beading, gathering, or subtle texturizing are the foxiest types of accents—as opposed to ruffles, feathers, and fur, which can look over the top.

It's essential to have a foxy wrap or shoulder throw for cool evenings—or just to give yourself a more glammed-up look. Choose a dressy silk cashmere or jacquard print, and you'll be swathed in style.

Fancify your feet in a pair of sexy sandals in cream, gold, or platinum gray. Look for something daring but comfortable, since you have to live in them all evening, through dinner, dancing, and possibly into the wee hours of the morning if it's really a swinging affair. For the best match, use this handy guide:

- **Black Dress:** black open-toe heels with black rhinestone detailing
- **Red Dress:** gold or taupe high-heel strappy sandals
- **Cream Dress:** platinum silk mule
- **Bronze Dress:** beige or gold beaded open-toe heel
- **Chiffon Dress:** strappy metallic sandals
- **Lace Dress:** matte satin slingbacks.

If you start with a divine dress, jewelry should be stunning and unfussy. Your goal is to accent, not overwhelm. You can't go wrong with diamonds—or good-looking sparkly knockoffs. A choker or graceful pendant, a set of studs or small dangle earrings, and a delicate bracelet draped over one wrist are all you need.

Finish off your formal look with an equally formal bag, such as a satin clutch with a rhinestone clasp, or a metallic mesh wrist purse. For added interest, it's best to choose a color that coordinates with but doesn't match your dress. And speaking of interest, don't be surprised if a few jaws drop as you make your enchanted entrance!

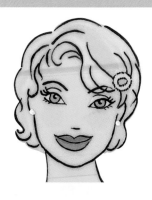

~Foxy Hair~

For a foxy formal, splurge on a salon blow out or fancy updo if you have the time. In thirty minutes, a good stylist can create something soft and sexy for any length hair. It'll save you hours of wrestling with bobby pins and Velcro curlers in an attempt to do it on your own. Take along a picture of a style you like from a magazine, but make sure it's something you'll be comfortable in all evening, and that it won't lose its shape the first time you get dipped on the dance floor.

You can also whip up a great look at home. Leave long hair flowing and natural rather than messing with a cumbersome up-do. Use a heavier than usual dose of volumizer and a jumbo brush to give the ends of your hair extra flip. For medium-length hair, try a half-up/half-down style. Blow your hair dry, pull the top portions back loosely, and clip them with small rhinestone, gold, or silver clips.

If you have shorter hair, put in a half-dozen small Velcro curlers before doing your makeup. Then remove the curlers and use shimmery hair wax to arrange the curls in piecey chunks and wisps. For a girly look, try a tiny sparkly vintage-style barrette on one side. You'll shine in more ways than one!

~Foxy Face and Bod~

Make sure your bod gets the black-tie treatment as well. Since you'll be baring a lot of skin in that sexy gown, give yourself an at-home tan a few days before the event, or get one at a salon.

With a golden glow as your base, layer on the Foxy Five. Foxify your eyes with shimmery beige or neutral pearl eye shadow. If you want more color, go with rose, plum, or soft gray tones rather than colors like blue and green, which can get you into trouble. For extra-plump lashes, use a volumizing mascara and apply two coats. It's easier and more foolproof than fake.

Finish off with a sophisticated fragrance; a soft floral is just the thing for such an elegant evening. To get the right amount, use a perfumed body lotion. After you've swathed your body, run your hands over your hair, and you'll be smelling foxy from head to toe.

Beware: With a look this foxy, you may suddenly start receiving a lot more invitations, so clear your calendar!

~Frumpy Fashion~

Sure, weddings are a time for "something old, something borrowed . . . " but that doesn't necessarily apply to wardrobe. Remember, this is someone's special once-in-a-lifetime day, so dress accordingly.

Divorce yourself from that slightly see-through linen skirt that wrinkles after you've had it on for five minutes, and puckers around your rear because it doesn't quite fit right. Same for that girlish flowered blouse that was snug and sexy last year but now looks a size too small. Disheveled duds may leave you looking like a flower child, rather than a flower girl.

From this day forward, vow to rid yourself of that blue suede miniskirt and the high-neck ruffled polyester blouse that looks like it's frothing up so much it's going to swallow you up. Unless it's a Vegas wedding with an Elvis theme, save the blue suede for a less formal affair—don't be cruel!

Be sure not to leave everyone with a case of wedding bell blues by wearing the wrong color. All black for a day wedding is just plain depressing, but a color that's too loud can be just as bad. The bride probably doesn't want you to be the bright neon blob that sticks out in every picture. There are plenty of occasions to pour on the vibrant colors, but for a day wedding, subtle shades should help ensure good placement in the photo album.

Hats are a foxy fave for wedding days, but the wrong one can leave you heading right back up the aisle. A rustic straw hat may give your beach look a boost, but it's too laid-back for this romantic rendezvous. And this probably isn't the best time to top off your look with that vintage oversized hand-me-down from Aunt Ruby—the floral accents and dramatic veil will just put you in competition with the bride.

Other than being there, one of the best gifts you can give to the happy couple is being a foxy friend. So when they recite "for better or for worse," let's make sure you're part of the better half.

~Frumpy Face and Bod~

If the heat and humidity are rising, so will the beads of perspiration on your foxy brows. Instead of tears of joy, you'll be shedding streams of sweat. The June bride may be "glowing," but you could end up giving the word new meaning.

Guest: Day

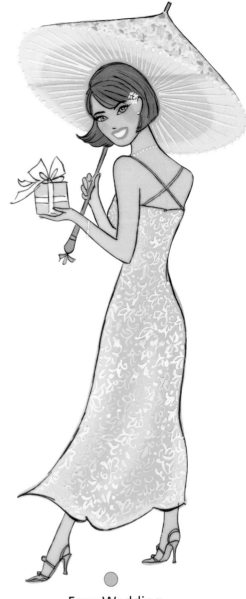

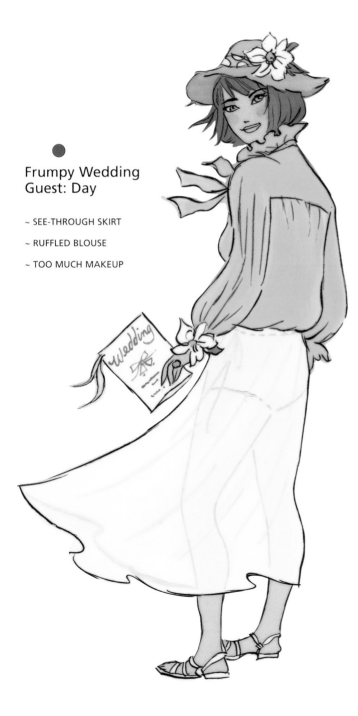

Frumpy Wedding Guest: Day

~ SEE-THROUGH SKIRT

~ RUFFLED BLOUSE

~ TOO MUCH MAKEUP

Foxy Wedding Guest: Day

~ HAIR PINNED BACK NEATLY

~ BREEZY, SILKY DRESS

~ SIMPLE, ELEGANT JEWELRY

Frumpy to Foxy in 15 Minutes ◔

~Foxy Fashion~

Just say I do, Foxy!

You don't need a license to create a blissful look for a summery day wedding. Slip into a breezy silk or chiffon tea-length dress in happy colors like pale yellow, light green, or a delicate floral print. Then add a coordinating slingback heel, equally good for sashaying down the aisle and spinning on the dance floor.

Catch the bouquet in a look to match: a flowing knee-length chiffon skirt with a silky flutter-sleeve top in floral colors like rose, lilac, or sweet pea. A strappy silk or leather sandal will carry you right over the threshold.

A bouclé skirt suit in soft pastel shades like peach, lime, or butter yellow will capture the mood of the afternoon. Tuck a cream-colored silk camisole underneath,

and dance the day away in matching or cream-colored peep-toes.

For a more casual outdoor wedding, a strapless sundress in a subtle floral or embroidered cotton is the perfect blend of dreamy and dressed-up. Finish off with mid-high heels so you don't wind up sinking into the grass . . . keep your foxy footing and you'll be swinging the night away under the stars.

The icing on the cake is a crushable wide-brimmed straw hat to keep the rice from sticking in your hair, and keep the sun from turning you the same blush pink as the roses.

For summer weddings when the romance is heating up, a few foxy accessories will help keep you cool. Tuck a floral paper fan into a straw handbag or clasped clutch.

And if the ceremony or reception is outside, a small silk parasol or Asian-style umbrella will "veil" you from the sun. It's the perfect way to celebrate a perfect day.

Finish off your look with a dainty pendant or solitaire diamond on a strand, and small dangle earrings to match. No need to pile on the bling, since the bride's jewels are the shining stars of this celebration.

Take these simple style secrets to have and to hold, and I now pronounce you foxy!

~Foxy Hair~

Tuck a few strands of baby's breath behind your ear or into your hair if you're wearing it up. And for heaven's sake if the weather's hot, please do wear it up! A formal up-do may be going overboard, but a simple bun will look classy and keep you cool. If the humidity is making you feel as though you stuck your finger in an electric socket, spend the money on a high-quality anti-frizz serum— it's worth it!

~Foxy Face and Bod~

Foxify your face with the sheer version of the Foxy Five, including a pale seashell pink blush and glistening neutral lip gloss. It's also a good idea to use clear mascara, and of course, clear deodorant. When choosing an appropriate fragrance, go for something light that won't overpower the guests at your table. Subtly foxy is the impression you want to make.

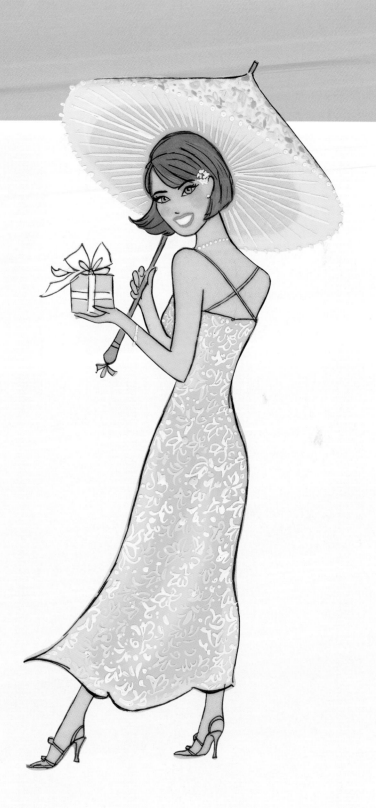

Frumpy to Foxy Wedding

~Frumpy Fashion~

Get the champagne ready: Two lovebirds are about to exchange their vows. Of course, when it comes to getting dressed, there are several ways to "trip" down the aisle as you find your way to your seat.

If there's one thing that's absolutely off-limits for an evening wedding guest, it's white. On the big day, there's only one person who should wear all white, and that's the bride! You'll know exactly why all eyes are on you while waiting in line for a piece of that irresistible banana cream wedding cake.

Just as the bride spent weeks, even months, before deciding on a dress, you should also give some thoughtful consideration to your attire. Wearing a tailored long-sleeve blouse and slacks just doesn't make the cut, even if you jazz it up with heels and pearls. You won't be doing any justice to the wedding photos with an outfit like that.

A wedding is an evening of elegance and class and the perfect reason to slip into our most dazzling duds, so short skirts or minis are off-limits. They're more appropriate for a night out on the town than a night of nuptials.

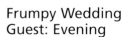

Frumpy Wedding Guest: Evening

~ WHITE OUTFIT

~ MINI-SKIRT

~ TOO MUCH GLITTER
  AND MAKEUP

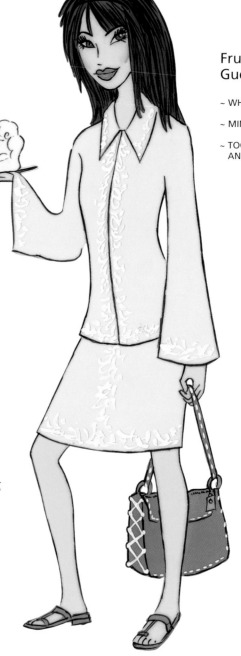

Guest: Evening

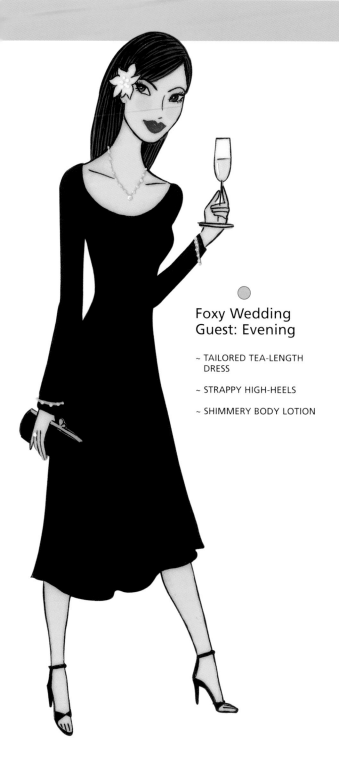

**Foxy Wedding
Guest: Evening**

~ TAILORED TEA-LENGTH
   DRESS

~ STRAPPY HIGH-HEELS

~ SHIMMERY BODY LOTION

Unless it's a wedding very close to or on the beach, flat thong sandals are also a big no-no. Reach for those when you're taking a weekend stroll.

Just in case there's any question: Don't even consider wearing jeans to a wedding, no matter what style they are. The bride and groom deserve something fancier than that.

~Frumpy Face and Bod~

If you're looking for the ultimate opportunity to get glam, an evening wedding is definitely it. With all of that love in the air, it would be a shame to do anything less. You don't want to show up looking like you fell face forward into the frumps—limp, lifeless hair and all.

If you're not going to splurge on a fancy do, then try something with a little more pizzazz than your typical nine-to-five office style. Now's the time to do it!

Even though it's tempting, veering way off in the other direction can be gawk-worthy as well, so it's best to stay away from wrapping your hair up into a big bouffant or tower of tresses. As the other guests start to get a bit tipsy, they may be tempted to poke at it all night long. Who could resist?

~Foxy Fashion~

Here comes the foxy! Break out that drop-dead dress—it's time to celebrate! The bride will be most appreciative of your foxiness.

Say "I do" to a tea-length dress in a fluid fabric and a rich color like emerald green, magenta, deep blue, dark silver, or black. Whether it's spaghetti strap, tank, short sleeve with a V-neck, or a round-neck full sleeve, you'll step right into the spirit of the evening in something long and luxurious. With the right pair of shoes, it's a match made in heaven:

- **Emerald Green or Magenta Dress:** black or gunmetal metallic and metal mesh evening bag

- **Deep Blue Dress:** black or silver strappy heels with a satin clutch

- **Dark Silver Dress:** black or matte satin gray mule with sequin clutch

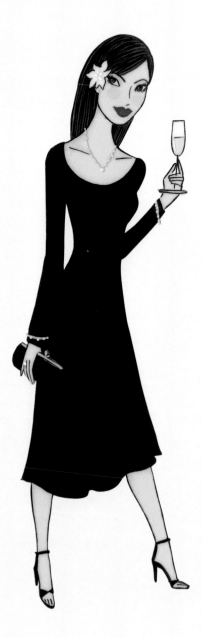

- **Black Dress:** platinum or deep red leather strappy high heels and and black wrist pouch

Stockings aren't a must for matrimonial affairs, but if you can't imagine not wearing hose, make sure you go super sheer with a closed-toe shoe.

For something a little slinkier, show up in an all-black ensemble: a lacy, halter-neck top (roomy enough to wiggle in) paired with a shin-length, silky skirt and black, high-heel Mary Janes. If you're not spoken for already, be prepared to catch the eyes of more than a few.

Pack a small beaded bag with all of the evening's essentials, and then add a few dazzling jewels (it doesn't matter if they're real or faux as long as they look foxy): diamond studs, a few diamond bangles, and a chunky semiprecious stone necklace (in amethyst, citrine, or garnet). The only thing left to do is blow a kiss to the bride.

~Foxy Hair~

For longer hair, try wrapping hair up in a loose chignon, or just pulling back the top, leaving the bottom loose and flowing. An evening wedding is a chance to try a romantic, touchable hairstyle. For shorter locks, use a pomade with a little shimmer to shape hair and also add a little something. No matter what length your hair is, fasten a flower (gardenia, orchid, or rose) behind your ear with a bobby pin. Now that's romance!

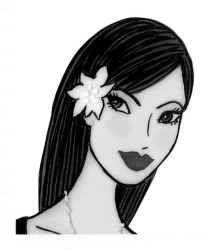

~Foxy Face and Bod~

Let everyone see the twinkle in your eyes as you toast the newlyweds. And get the hankies ready, since you may be shedding a few tears of joy. Let's make sure that makeup doesn't smear off along the way! Getting ready for an evening wedding is as easy as sticking to your everyday makeup routine, but with a twist. Go for a light eye and dramatic lip effect by adding sheer, off-white shimmer shadow to your lids and above your cheekbones. If you have one, use an eyelash curler to lengthen and spread your lashes out. Fatten those lashes with extra mascara. Better yet, make that waterproof mascara to prevent any black, runny gunk from streaming down your face during the emotional exchanging of vows.

Sure, there will be flowers, but make your lips your very own centerpiece for the night. Drench them in a deep red or pinkish brown color to really turn them out. Add a bit of matching lip liner for extra definition and wow. Unfortunately for the other guests, this is one centerpiece they won't be taking home.

Before donning your duds, cover your arms, neck, and shoulders in a shimmering body lotion. That means soft, velvety skin with a touch of added glow all in one quick swipe. Now that's living happily ever after!

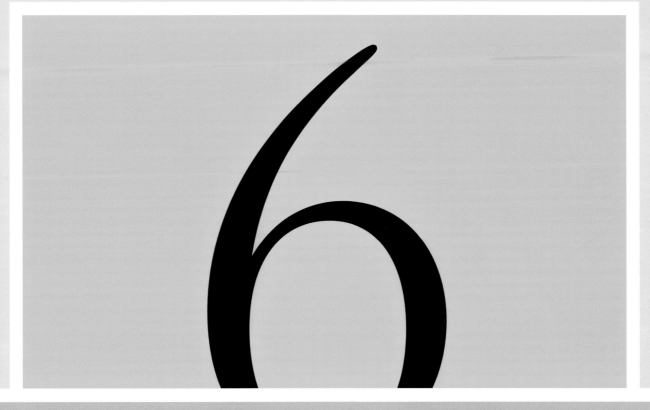

6

Foxy On the Go

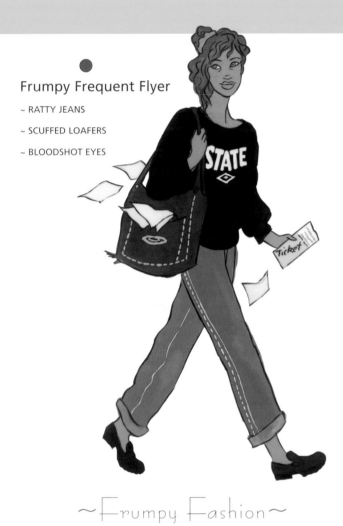

Frumpy Frequent Flyer

~ RATTY JEANS

~ SCUFFED LOAFERS

~ BLOODSHOT EYES

~Frumpy Fashion~

As we climb that corporate ladder, we may have to take our show on the road from time to time, but that doesn't mean leaving our sense of style at home. The pressures of long, cramped flights, frantic airport shuffles, and suitcase dynamics can lead us to the wrong fashion choices and leave us flying the frumpy skies instead of the friendly skies.

The business staple is the suit, but the wrong suit can make the wrong impression. To play it stylishly safe, avoid pleated suit pants, bulky shoulders, and suit jackets longer than your upper thigh. After all, you're a career girl, not a career pilot. Faded oxford shirts with button-down collars are a look that says outdated, not outstanding. And don't count on the fact that hiding a sweat-stained polyester shell underneath that suit jacket will camouflage the quality.

Flying can be a less-than-foxy experience, but that doesn't mean it should be frumpy. There's always a chance you'll bump into acquaintances or coworkers on your flight, and you don't want them to catch you in ratty jeans and a sweatshirt. Talk about needing an upgrade! Even executive privilege won't buy you a stamp of approval on that.

One of the trickiest traps for traveling gals is the "comfortable shoe." Sure, our dainty feet swell when we fly, and we've all had to do the mad dash from Terminal C to Terminal H to catch that connector flight, but scuffed loafers and flats with a worn-down lopsided heel look like cattle class, not first class.

The vinyl computer case with the big logo that one of your "valued clients" sent you definitely isn't the best choice of briefcase. Not only does it have zero style, but everyone will know you got it as a freebie, so wave it good-bye before you board.

Frequent Flyer

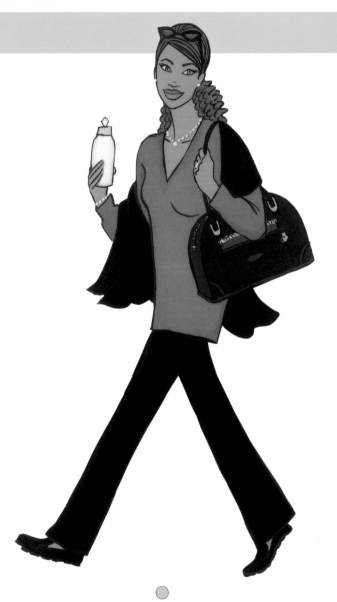

Foxy Frequent Flyer

~ BLACK COTTON KNIT PANTS

~ LEATHER CARRY-ON BAG

~ BOTTLED WATER TO STAY HYDRATED

~Frumpy Face and Bod~

Travel is tough on our feminine facades, and we have to work extra hard not to succumb to the frequent flier frumps.

Flying does wicked things to our skin, hair, and eyes, and after a five-hour flight, we can end up looking like the Bride of Frankenstein's scary stepsister. Chapped lips, faded skin, bloodshot eyes, frizzy hair and all. And if that isn't scary enough, the awful lighting in airplane lavatories turns frumpy into downright frightening.

There's no need to doll yourself up for the plane ride; you'll only end up looking "undone" by the time the plane touches down. A face full of makeup will not make you look rested and rosy at the end of the flight; instead, you'll end up looking smudged, smattered, and caked-on. And that fancy hairdo you worked so hard to perfect will look smashed—or like you flew in on a broomstick.

Once you've reached your destination, it's best not to rely on hotel mini-soaps and shampoos, which can be full of drying ingredients. Same for those handy-dandy wall-mounted hair dryers—turns out they aren't quite so handy or dandy. They've been known to fry, entangle, and otherwise torture our luscious locks, so place the "do not disturb" sign on those.

Frumpy to Foxy in 15 Minutes 🕐

~Foxy Fashion~

Move on up to first class, Foxy! A few simple tricks can ensure fashionable frequent flying whether you travel once a year or once a month.

The essential in-flight outfit is a pair of full-length stretchy black cotton or knit pants with a wide leg, paired with a shapely hip-length V-neck sweater and super-soft driving loafers (they've got more give to pamper your puffy feet). This is the closest thing we've found to traveling in our pj's, and it looks fresh and foxy whether we're deplaning in London or Las Vegas. Be sure to pack a wrap for the plane; a black wrap in silk cashmere or wool keeps us cozy warm in that chilly climate-controlled cabin, and doubles as a scarf on winter trips—a foxy two-in-one!

Whether you're on your way to power meetings, an important presentation, or a crowded convention, a few foxy fundamentals are all you need. The number one must-have is a classic suit with a flared pant and tailored jacket that hits at the hip, in chocolate brown, tan, or black. It can be dressed up or down, goes with any color on Earth, and doesn't show dirt—a foxy three-in-one!

Pack a trio of tops that can be mixed, matched, and layered: a colored V-neck sweater in cotton or a cashmere blend, a coordinating pattern blouse, and a crisp white button-down. If your trip is more than a few days, add a silk tank or cashmere turtleneck and an extra fitted blazer in a neutral tan.

Shoes should be comfortable and classy; walkable black pumps, high-heel loafers, or black low-heel ankle boots will work through the day and into dinner. Pack some sheer trouser socks as well.

Keep jewelry simple when you're traveling. All you need is pearl earrings and a set of studs, a silver pendant, and a watch to keep you in the right time zone.

A structured leather bag will hold all your in-flight essentials, and that extra pack of pretzels that you're saving for later. And don't forget those foxy details, such as an organizer or hip notepad and a sleek silver or black pen for jotting notes during those networking sessions—much cooler than using a cocktail napkin!

If you're tired and weary-eyed upon arrival and it's still light out, have a pair of sunglasses on hand . . . even if the paparazzi aren't waiting for you.

~Foxy Hair~

Hair care doesn't have to be high maintenance: Simply pack a replenishing hair conditioner and gloss to tame post-flight frizzies. If you're bonded at the hip to your blow-dryer, bring along a travel dryer with adjustable heat settings. A compact curling iron and a black hair clip are other trusty take-alongs that will keep your tresses traveling well, instead of looking well-traveled.

~Foxy Face and Bod~

The key to preserving a foxy face on the road can be summed up in one word: hydration! A girl's best friend is moisturizer; use a heavier one than normal to combat the arid airplane atmosphere. And keep in mind that hotel air isn't much better.

To keep ourselves foxified in flight and afterward, we never leave home without a tube of lip balm, purse-size hand lotion, moisturizing eye drops, and a small spray bottle of facial mist.

Before arriving at your gate, soothe your skin with a smothering of Elizabeth Arden 8-Hour Cream, or any other ultra-rich moisturizer.

Your makeup can be minimal but should also be geared toward moisturizing your mug. Try a creamier foundation and apply it with a slightly wet sponge to ensure dewy skin. Replace your usual blush with a subtle bronzer to give yourself extra sunny color. Add cover-up to camouflage those jet-lag circles, a curl of your lashes to give your eyes that rested and ready look, and a quick coat of mascara, and you've got a ticket to ride!

Last but not least, the number one gotta-have-it on-the-go essential is good ol' H_2O. Drink it like it's going out of style, and it will keep you in style. It's like a fresh, foxy face in a bottle, so guzzle up.

Foxy Tip: When packing, roll your clothes instead of folding them. You'll prevent wrinkles!

Frumpy to Foxy Vacation:

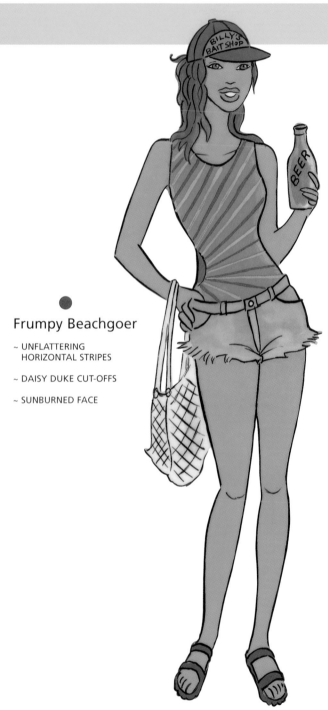

Frumpy Beachgoer

~ UNFLATTERING
  HORIZONTAL STRIPES

~ DAISY DUKE CUT-OFFS

~ SUNBURNED FACE

~Frumpy Fashion~

There's nothing like the warm, wonderful glow you get from a week in the tropics: lounging seaside with a mai-tai in hand, barefoot romps in the sand, cooling dips in the water. Nothing could be finer— and nothing could be frumpier if you don't pack the right gear!

Bathing suits never look on mortal humans the way they look on supermodels. Whether the bulge is in the stomach or the derriere, whether you're hippy or flat as a board, wearing a bathing suit can seem like a cruel joke of Mother Nature. She didn't really intend for anyone to look good in that itsy-bitsy, teeny-weeny bikini, did she?

Frumpy swimsuit mishaps are almost too many to count. First, there's fit. If it's too small, it will ride up your bottom, won't contain your breasts, or will show too much of everything. If it's too big, you'll look like a poor hand-me-down.

The wrong pattern and color can also sabotage your foxiness. Stripes may work on a prison uniform, but

Beach

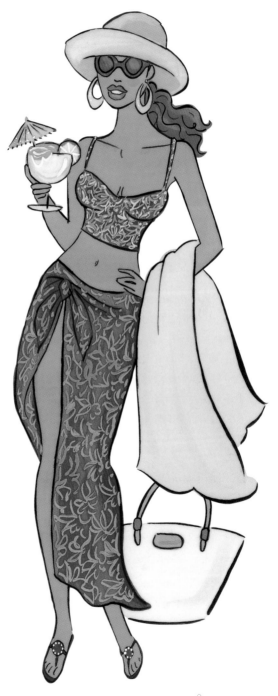

on a swimsuit they can accentuate all the wrong things. Horizontals can give you that beached bumblebee look, and vertical can leave you looking like an NFL ref. Neons and fluorescents will have you glowing in the dark long after you've left the pool. They may look summery in the store, but don them in broad daylight, and you could find yourself swimming in a sea of glowfish. White can be equally dangerous; if it's not lined properly, you could be sharing a little more than you bargained for with your fellow sunbathers.

Make sure you have the right cover-up for the pool. That doesn't mean a knee-length "tress" (a T-shirt big enough to be a dress). And those denim cutoffs that inch up your thighs every year will soon be technically a "bikini bottom." The old baseball cap that advertises BILLY'S BAIT SHOP may get you thrown into the pool by a local fisherman, but won't win you any foxy points either.

Beach vacations are the ultimate, but not if you end up looking like a beach bum.

~Frumpy Face and Bod~

The brochure for that tropical beach getaway featured a gorgeous girl on the front with a killer tan and windswept hair, so why is it that we end up looking like someone spray painted our bodies with red dye number 13? This is one time when it's not cool to "feel the burn." Not covering up with sunscreen could leave you with a nasty case of lobster face or farmer's tan, which will then be

Frumpy to Foxy in 15 Minutes ⏱

~Foxy Fashion~

Hang ten, Foxy! Whether you're headed for an afternoon at a local beach or off for a glorious week-long holiday in an exotic locale, start with a good swimsuit. Not sure what style suits your shape? When in doubt, choose a one piece or tankini—not a tiny triangle of cloth connected by two pieces of thread.

Check for full butt and breast coverage. It's a good idea to take a friend along when you try on suits so you don't have to rely on those awful mirrors; they can make you want to run and hide that pale, ghostly body underneath several layers of nuclear-proof garb.

Look "see-worthy" in the right style for your shape:

- If you're straight as a surfboard, try a belted suit to give you a waistline.
- If you have short legs, a higher-cut bottom makes legs look longer.
- If you want to hide your belly, look for a ruched one piece.
- If you want to minimize large breasts, choose an athletic two-piece or medium-neck tank.
- If you want to supersize small breasts, sport a lighter halter top with darker bottoms.

Foxy Tip: If you're not comfortable in a swimsuit, a tropical-inspired backup is board shorts and a tummy-covering tank.

Swimsuits are like jeans: It's hard to find one that fits, so when you do, grab at least one, or buy two in different colors. Flattering swimsuit colors are black, navy, red, or a bronzy brown, but stick with colors that you know work best on you. Keep skin tone in mind, pre- and post-tan. You want a color that accentuates the positive whether you're pale or golden. Delicate floral prints and textures can work well, but stick with darker shades.

For lounging poolside, toss on a terry mini or knee-length stretchy skirt and a zip-up hoodie. For a more tropical foxy look, try a sarong combined with a fitted tank. One of the comfiest après-swim looks is a slightly loose-fitting tank tee dress—for that quick jaunt to the souvenir shop.

followed by dry, peeling swatches of skin and unsightly sweat bumps. We're pretty sure that wasn't in the brochure. Salt water can wreak havoc, too, leaving hair matted and mussed.

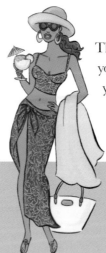

The laid-back vibe of the tropics can persuade you to feel a bit too lax about your looks, leaving you with scaly skin, parched lips, and frazzled hair. But it should be the opposite—it's easy to look foxy while having fun in the sun.

There's only one way to go with shoes at the beach: When you're not barefoot, just don bold-colored flip-flops or plastic slides. They're perfect for sand, street, or local outdoor café.

For dressier beachside evenings, throw on a cotton halter or strapless tube dress in white, lime, black, or turquoise. Then add flat grommeted leather sandals that you can kick off for those starry strolls along the water. Equally foxy are light cotton or linen palazzo pants with a relaxed tank sweater over a camisole. Finish off with flat braided sandals and a chunky choker around your bronzed neckline.

The must-have foxy accessories for any tropical trip are a wide-brimmed straw hat to protect your foxy face, sunglasses, and a brightly colored striped or patterned beach tote and towel. An orange-hued towel reflects the warm tones in your foxy face.

~Foxy Hair~

Take along a bottle of hair spritz to protect those locks from the elements. A leave-in conditioner or "beach hair" spray with a yummy scent and a little salt will give you natural sea-swept curls.

Or sweep longer hair into a tropical knot. Make a low braid, secure with an elastic, wind the braid around itself a few times, and tie at your nape. If your hair's short, just twist it. You'll look refreshingly foxy for those ocean-side afternoons.

~Foxy Face and Bod~

No foxette would be caught dead lying out in the sun without sunscreen. It's a must to protect that lovely skin, whether you're fair or olive. Make sure to slather your whole bod in it, from head to toe. To help lips stay as supple as a slice of mango, keep them coated in a coconut-scented lip balm with sunscreen. Slather on an aloe vera gel after basking on the beach all day to cool your skin and help prevent it from peeling.

Our final foxy beach staple is body oil. Spritz throughout the day and give yourself a glowing, rather than "dried up raisin," look. Surf's up, Foxy!

Frumpy to Foxy Vacation:

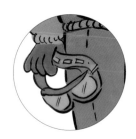

~Frumpy Fashion~

Baby it's cold outside, so make sure you're dressed like one hot babe.

A mistake we've all made is just too many darn layers. They may keep us toasty warm, but can also leave us looking like we packed on a few pounds overnight. Brrrr!

Another frump-trap: a love affair with plaid flannel. Plaid can be charming and cute in a schoolgirl kind of way, but it's not the right look for a foxified frosty getaway. Somehow it always looks like you're wearing pj's, and it's tough to make a plaid flannel shirt look foxy.

Same for those dependable thermal cotton undies. They served their purpose again and again, but it's time to say so long to long johns. With the saggy rear and rustic waffle pattern, they could make you look a little too much like the local park ranger.

A final word of caution before kicking up some powder: Don't go with one color from head to toe in an effort to be the most stylish snow bunny on the slopes. An overdose of pink and you really *will* look like a bunny; too much green and you could look like a super-size Shrek flying down the mountain.

You're not suiting up for a Siberian winter, so there's no need for an oversized hunter's hat that keeps flapping over your eyes. As you're whizzing down the slopes, you don't want to bowl down other skiers and boarders on the way.

~Frumpy Face and Bod~

As fun as a cold-weather vacation can be, after being exposed to the sun, wind, and sub-zero temps, you can come home feeling like the icewoman. There's something not quite so appealing about chapped lips, blue hands, swollen feet, and a runny nose.

And after a day on the slopes, you might find out that cozy ski-cap has left you with a permanent dose of really bad hat hair. Time to call in the ski patrol!

Skiing

Frumpy Skier

~ OVERDOSE OF ONE COLOR

~ OVERSIZED HUNTER'S HAT

~ A BAD CASE OF HAT HAIR

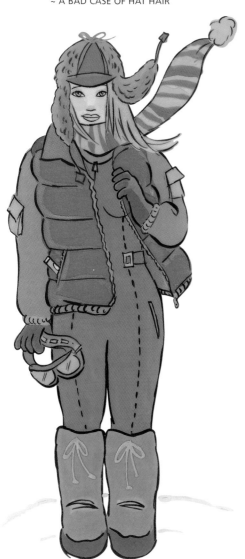

Foxy Skier

~ STRETCHY SKI PANTS
  WITH A STIRRUP BOTTOM

~ FLEECE-LINED LACE-UP BOOTS

~ SLEEK WOOL CAP

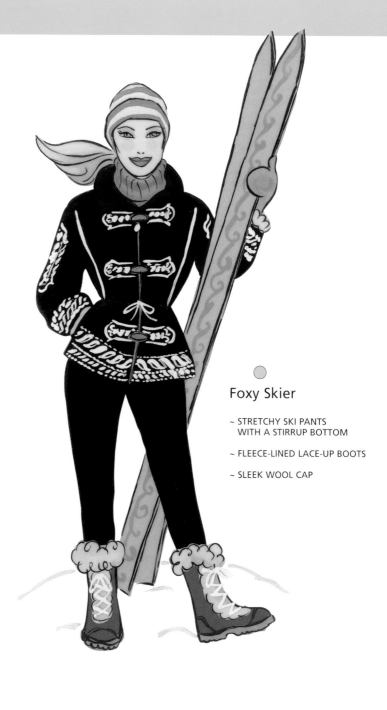

foxy on the go 125

~Foxy Fashion~

Let it snow, Foxy!

Hit the lifts in stretchy black ski pants with stirrup bottoms. The stirrups pull the pants down, creating a straight line instead of a bunchy mess, so you look slim instead of snowman-esque. Underneath, wear silk long johns; they'll give you that extra layer of insulation without all the bulk.

Layering your upper half is a bit more involved. Depending on temperatures and wind chill, you might need two layers or more. Start with a silk tank, then a long-sleeve silk T-shirt; both provide insulation but wick away moisture if you start to overheat from all that swooshin' and slidin'. Follow with a medium-weight zip-up cotton Lycra top in a bold color—pink, red, or sailing yellow. If you need an extra layer, make it a chunky wool turtleneck sweater in black.

Cap it all off with a brightly colored ski jacket that's belted or cinched at the waist, which not only keeps snow from getting under your clothing but also slims your look. The most flattering length hits at the hip. The key, as always, is functionality = foxiness.

Another foxy look is blue or cream snowboard pants. They're warm and padded, but more flattering than traditional puffy ski pants. Snowboard gear has straighter unisex lines that look sporty and slimming. Go with a coordinating snowboard jacket, and you'll slide and glide in style.

Take along some serious black ski socks with a thinner sock to layer underneath.

Foxy Tip: If you're a foxette with fragile feet, buy a few thermal heat packets and stick them in your boots when you suit up. They'll keep your feet from getting that frostbite feel.

Your look off the slopes is just as important. Our favorite time is après ski, sipping hot chocolate and snuggling up with a significant other. Fire things up with stretchy brown or plum flared-leg pants in thick cotton. Combine them with a thigh-length cream-colored cable-knit sweater and cozy brown suede driving loafers or cushiony fleece-lined lace-up boots.

If you're going out for a walk in the midnight snow, throw on some boots with a rugged sole, and a long shearling coat. Protect your head and hands with black or brown gloves, a matching scarf, and a small colored wool cap—nothing with fringe or pompoms. Keep it simple, Foxy, and you'll be stylin' from the lifts to the lodge.

~Foxy Hair~

No matter how cool we look coming down that double black diamond, we get to the bottom, remove our caps, and end up with a matted, rumpled mess of hat hair. To keep their tresses on the trail, gals with medium-length or long hair should spray their locks with protective leave-in conditioner and slick it back into a ponytail. Gals with short hair should use a moisturizing gel and do the same. The hat is going to plaster your hair anyway, so you might as well beat it to the punch and start with a slicked back do.

Cold-weather trips are also a good time to use a heavier conditioner than normal. Try something with milk protein or olive oil, and your hair will look like it vacationed in St. Tropez, not St. Moritz.

~Foxy Face and Bod~

While chapped lips may not be totally unavoidable in cold, windy weather, you can do your best to combat the elements with a tube of industrial-strength lip balm. Choose something with emollients and sunscreen; it'll moisturize and protect your smackers from sun and wind.

Treat your hands just as delicately. Use the heaviest moisturizer you can find to fight the frost. Cover every inch of your body in sunscreen every morning before you hit the slopes; otherwise, you'll end up with sunburn and very unattractive goggle lines around your eyes—Rocky Raccoon! Because you're cold when you ski, you might not realize how much sun you're getting. And don't forget that you're at higher altitudes where you get extra exposure. So lube up before you luge.

Foxy Tip: Take along a small pack of travel tissues, since cold weather can leave you with an annoyingly runny nose. And stick a tube of Vaseline in your pocket. You can use it on your hands and lips, to tame hair frizzies, and even to calm the occasional blisters you get from skiing too hard.

Frumpy to Foxy Vacation:

~Frumpy Fashion~

Wandering the cobblestone streets of Rome, peering through the gates of Buckingham Palace, and snapping photos from atop the Eiffel Tower in Paris can be unforgettable.

So can prancing into a bustling sidewalk café in Barcelona wearing your puffy Bermuda shorts, golf shirt, oversized backpack, and hippie sandals, while all of the well-heeled locals turn around to give you the once-over.

Your favorite college sweatshirt, black leggings, and baseball cap may be comfy for all-day sightseeing, but taking a cruise along the enchanting Seine calls for something other than clothing fit for a college basketball rally. If the French had a word for "frumpy," this would be it!

Food is one of the sweetest parts of any European getaway—sampling *fromage* or enjoying a buttery croissant and a glass of Chardonnay at a quaint café is something to savor forever. But doing it in head-to-toe tourist attire doesn't quite fit the picture, so say *au revoir* to the bright orange terrycloth visor, fanny pack, plaid shorts, blousy collared T-shirt, and sneakers with thick, bunchy white socks. And that bulky camera slung around your neck doesn't qualify as a fashion accessory. Not a pretty picture.

You may think a tracksuit is just the thing to wear while exploring the Louvre Museum, but with all of that unavoidable European sophistication oozing from every corner, it's definitely a faux pas. The Mona Lisa deserves more, and so do you, Foxy.

~Frumpy Face and Bod~

There's nothing like immersing yourself in the culture of a new, uncharted city. Wearing your hair in "Pippi Longstocking" braids for a trip to Sweden isn't the best way to do it.

Traveling to such fashionable cities as Milan and Berlin may tempt you to experiment with outrageous makeup colors you'd find strictly on the runways. But the black lipstick and cherry red eye shadow are better off on the models, not on you.

Even though some Europeans are fond of going au natural by not making regular use of a razor, that doesn't mean you should jump on the bandwagon. Beware of immersing yourself in the culture to the point where you have an inch of underarm hair blowing carelessly in the Riviera breeze. There are easier ways to experience and enjoy local customs, so keep things fuzz-free and find something else to write home about.

Europe

Frumpy European Vacationer

~ PLAID BERMUDA SHORTS

~ TERRY CLOTH VISOR
AND FANNY PACK

~ HEAVY SOCKS
AND SNEAKERS

Foxy European Vacationer

~ TAN CAPRIS

~ "JACKIE O"-STYLE
SUNGLASSES

~ PUCCI SCARF

Frumpy to Foxy in 15 Minutes ⊙

~Foxy Fashion~

Bellisima, Foxy! As they say, "When in Rome, do as the Romans do!" Pack your dapper duds and get ready to dine al fresco with a delicious bowl of pasta puttanesca.

There's only one way to take in all that European culture—on foot. Whether strolling the Champs Elysee or skipping down the Spanish Steps, foxettes know the secret to successful sightseeing: casual and classic ensembles will ensure that *you* are the sight to be seen. As usual, it's best to keep your look simple.

Breeze through the museums in a knee-length, black, fluid skirt with a colorful cotton T-shirt and slim sneakers. The Van Goghs, Monets, and Picassos look even more beautiful when you're gazing at them in comfort. Remember to wear very low socks, so you don't have anything peeking out above the lip of your sneaker. Leave the pom-pom socks at home, foxy!

Can't resist the urge to splurge on designer duds? Hit the shops in tan Capri pants, a short-sleeve white button-down shirt with a thin scarf around your neck, and cushiony ballet flats. Add some oversized "Jackie O"-style shades and a small nylon zippered tote, and you could easily be mistaken for a local.

An evening walk around the bustling city square is that much foxier when you're wearing black palazzo pants and an off-the-shoulder coordinating silk sweater with an open-toe, cork wedge sandal. Pair this look with some simple dangle earrings. If it gets chilly,

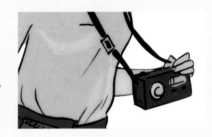

stay away from bulky coats that could make you look ready for the Arctic, not a night out. Instead, bring a soft, cashmere wrap with you. Très chic!

Slip into a halter-top sundress and grommeted sandals and you'll be ready to saunter through those quaint Mediterranean seaside villages and drink in the postcard-perfect sunsets in style. A small slim bag worn over the shoulder will store your necessities and keep your hands free for souvenir shopping.

Too much jewelry can immediately target you as a "tourista," so go easy on the baubles. A day-or-night pair of small hoops or dangles and a casual watch are the only accents you need to be understood in any language.

You've got the ticket to traveling in style, so whether the destination is Cannes or Cairo, show the world that you're a foreigner with flair.

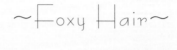

~Foxy Hair~

Pull long hair back in a ponytail with a Pucci-style scarf tied around it for irresistible European flair. If you have short hair, simply wrap the scarf around your head. You'll be all set for an afternoon of cruising the city on the back of a Vespa.

~Foxy Face and Bod~

When it comes to your face, avoid wild colors and stick with the Foxy Five. As for the rest of your body, don't forget to pack your trusty razor to keep stubble from growing like an enormous field of French lavender! For a night out, a small dab of just the right perfume will give you a certain *je ne sais quoi*.

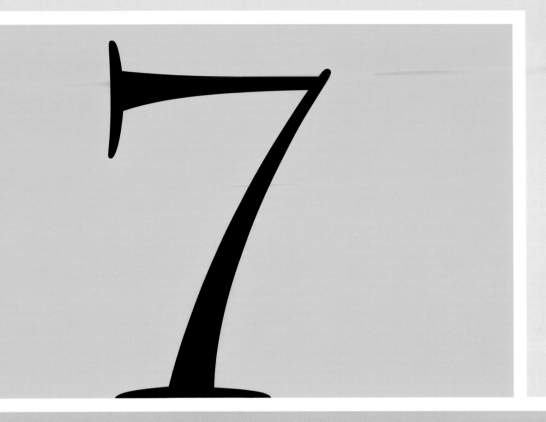

Foxy Family

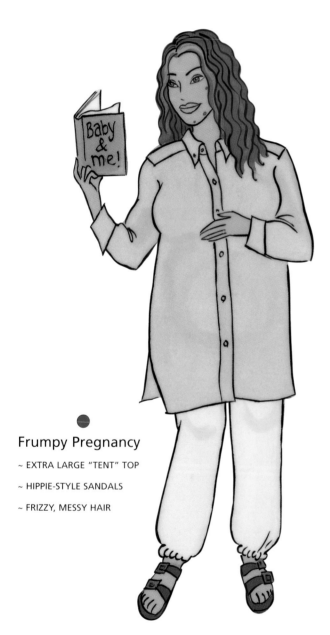

Frumpy Pregnancy

~ EXTRA LARGE "TENT" TOP

~ HIPPIE-STYLE SANDALS

~ FRIZZY, MESSY HAIR

~Frumpy Fashion~

If anytime's the right time to break out in the frumps, then pregnancy—with the accompanying swollen feet, morning sickness, an ever-expanding belly, and hips wide enough to fit into Shaquille O'Neal's basketball shorts—sure seems to be it.

Maternity clothes? Foxy? Sounds like a riddle for the sphinx. If full-length caftans, baggy farm-style overalls, and oversized boxy T-shirts with long cotton skirts sound familiar, then it's time to do some frump control.

Your husband's XL rugby shirt that's been hanging in the back of the closet for a few years coupled with a pair of supersized sweatpants isn't the answer either. As your tummy expands, it doesn't mean your tops have to turn into tents. Those giant Hawaiian-print button-downs left over from spring break might work better as tablecloths than as stylish tops over the next trimester.

As your feet puff out (and they will!), you may be tempted to try out some "alternative footwear" such as hippie-style sandals, but they belong in the frumpy hall of fame. There are definitely more stylish and comfortable options.

Pregnancy

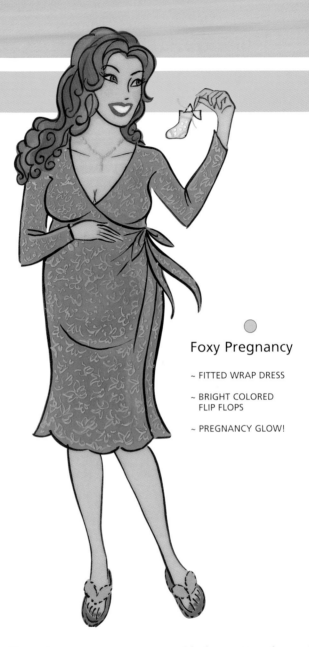

Foxy Pregnancy

~ FITTED WRAP DRESS

~ BRIGHT COLORED
   FLIP FLOPS

~ PREGNANCY GLOW!

These nine months aren't a time to hide under dumpy, dowdy duds. Start letting that big, beautiful belly bare itself a little more. Flaunt it, Foxy!

~Frumpy Face and Bod~

Who feels like getting foxified in the morning when all you can do is chew on crackers to get rid of the nausea? Pregnancy can be an emotional time, so all the more reason to keep yourself looking good.

When you're feeling rotten and Mother Nature's playing havoc with your system, the changes your body is going through may become visible in rather annoying ways. Your hair may be a frizzy, tangled mess, and you probably aren't planning on coloring it for a while. Alas, those feisty grays have popped out, and your hair starts to look more like a skunk tail.

You know it's time for a pick-me-up when you sneak a quick peek of yourself in the rearview mirror and realize you haven't seen your favorite lip gloss in days and you forgot what mascara looks like. Oh, baby . .

To make matters worse, your skin has gotten dry and flaky, and a bunch of funny-looking brown spots (an unfortunate perk of pregnancy) have suddenly found a comfortable place for themselves all over your face. Throw in some brand-new stretch marks and raging hormones, and it's time to call Foxy 911.

Frumpy to Foxy in 15 Minutes 🕐

~Foxy Fashion~

Let it all hang out, Foxy! Once upon a time it was fashionable to hide your body during pregnancy. Fortunately, things have changed. Time to embrace the bulge.

One of the best benefits of having a bun in the oven is that if you didn't have them before, you'll finally have buxom breasts, so a good bra is essential. True, it probably won't look like a lacy demi-cup out of some sexy lingerie catalog, but it doesn't have to look like your grandma's girdle either. It's possible to still feel foxy in a full-coverage style with a touch of lace.

Luckily, it's become much easier to find tasteful maternity clothes. And the good news is that there are a lot more options to explore while expecting: Tailored button-down shirts, A-line skirts, wrap dresses, bell-sleeve tops, and empire waists look flattering once your tummy starts to grow.

Stretchy tees show off your belly in the most becoming way, as do thigh-length V-neck sweaters. And since that little bun is going to grow for nine months, go ahead and invest in a good pair of contemporary maternity jeans and black slacks. Look for styles that have a stretchy waistline and a slightly longer leg, which helps lengthen the body. They will be your staples and help you resist the urge to return to the frumps. You'll look so foxy, your friends may even ask to borrow your clothes!

Strappy, high-heel sandals can be tough when you're pretty far along. Who wants thin heels when your ankles are getting thicker? Try a style with rubber soles and cushiony insteps that will give you much-needed padding while carrying the extra weight. You'll practically live in trusty sneakers or a cheerful pair of flip-flops with a padded sole during the warmer months—and even after you deliver the baby.

Before the stork arrives, put a little imagination into your maternity look and prepare to welcome your bundle of joy in style!

~Foxy Hair~

Hair, hair. Glorious, gorgeous, growing hair. Take advantage of those bountiful, bushy manes. All that extra shine can make hair easier to work with. What a relief! If, however, pregnancy is not pumping up the volume on your hair, and instead leaving it flat and frizzy, then pile on some pure cocoa butter conditioner for three minutes. Check out your health food store for something organic, since natural products are always a plus for expectant moms.

If the thought of spending nine months with gray or unsightly roots is rattling your nerves, chat with a pro about what you can do to get you through. Your stylist will be able to recommend a haircut or hair style that may minimize the need for coloring. There are also natural alternatives to coloring which may get the OK from the OB.

~Foxy Face and Bod~

Talk about having something to look forward to: Big beauty companies would hit the jackpot if they could capture that unmistakable pregnancy glow. It's a look no peel, cream, or makeup can match. At least it makes up for those months of morning sickness. And think about all the time you saved by not having to put anything more on your face than a tinted moisturizer with SPF, light blush,

and mascara. Keep a tinted lip balm nearby to add some moist color to your lips.

If your skin is extra flaky during those first few months, carry a rosewater or cucumber facial mist around with you, and load up with a heavy facial moisturizer at bedtime. As for those devilish brown blotches, a long-lasting cover-up like Amazing Concealer will hide them in no time. If anything worse than that pops up—like bad breakouts or a trail of brown spots—it's best to talk to the doc.

Foxy Tip: Make your own cucumber tonic at home by slicing up a cuke into a spray bottle of spring water. Sprinkle in a few drops of lavender oil for a calming touch.

Since stretch marks have a funny way of popping up all over the place, take a few minutes each morning and night to load up on

organic cocoa butter around your hips, tummy, and thighs.

Now that you're foxified, it's just how many months more 'til the stork arrives?

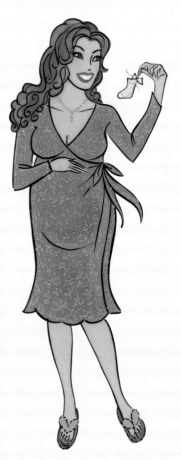

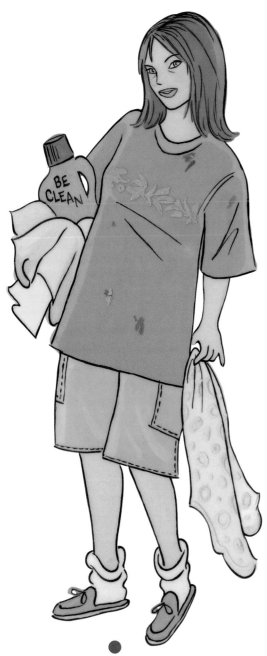

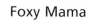

Foxy Mama

~ COMFORTABLE, BUT NOT
  TOO WORN JEANS

~ FUN, COLORFUL SNEAKERS

~ SHORT "WASH AND GO"
  HAIRCUT

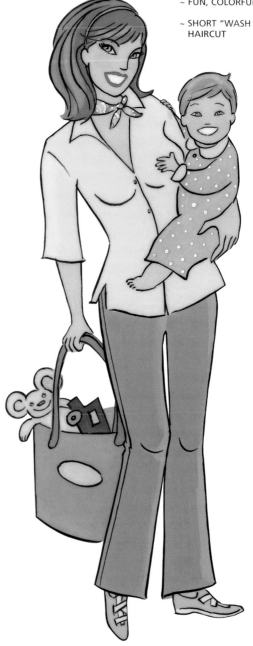

Frumpy Mama

~ STAINED, OLD T-SHIRT

~ BAGGY SHORTS

~ DARK ROOTS

Frumpy to Foxy: Mama

~Frumpy Fashion~

The number one frump trap in any woman's life is motherhood. Whether their kids are three or thirteen, moms always seem to fall into that old habit of saying, "I just don't have time." But it doesn't take a lot of time to dress like a foxy mama.

The first rule of parenthood: Don't try to dress like a teenager. Even if you have your pre-baby body back (more power to you!), the low-cut, belly-baring jeans and see-through tank just aren't great "mom" gear. Save the push up bra for a night out with your sweetie; it's probably not the right choice for the PTA meeting or that meeting with the principal.

And if you have toddlers, anything white is risky at best. Let's face it, by noon you'll look like an abstract painting with various shades of pea-green, grape-juice purple, and muddy brown smeared all over you.

But that doesn't mean you should wave the white flag of surrender and submit yourself to a uniform of faded gray sweatpants and sweatshirt, or baggy knee-length shorts and a kid-proof tattered T-shirt, which is often the last-gasp effort for many over-worked and underslept mamas.

Kids are cute, quirky, energetic, and a zillion other things, but they're not always clean, and as a mom, you have to be dressed for battle, not for afternoon tea. So leave the flowery gauzy skirt and barely-there silk cami for another occasion—maybe after your kids have graduated from college! If you have a baby or toddler, steer clear of long, dangle earrings. They're irresistible to little ones who just want to reach up and pull.

~Frumpy Face and Bod~

Between soccer practice, ballet lessons, play dates, slumber parties, school meetings, and the overkill of other kid-oriented activities, who has time to get her hair done? Gone are the days of supremely coiffed TV supermoms; today's mom is more likely to look like a frazzled woman with faded skin and dark circles under her eyes.

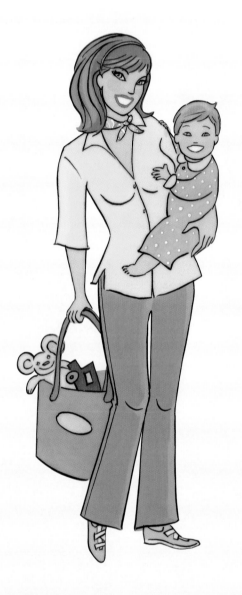

~Foxy Fashion~

Hey there, Foxy Mama! Teach those youngsters how to dress with the perfect combination of homespun practicality and "hot mama" panache.

There's no way to make it through parenthood without a foxy pair of jeans. If you find a style you like, buy them in bulk. Childbearing can take a toll on our hips, so we love a pair of medium-wash denims that are tailored but not too tight. Make sure they're not too short, either, since high-waters aren't so foxy. Wear them with a crisp, colorful, three-quarter-sleeve blouse (pinks, reds, and pale yellows are pretty and flattering). And finish off with a pair of suede loafers or feminine-but-flexible flats with cushy soles.

Another mom staple is a pair of flat-front capri-length khakis paired with layered tees in plummy earth tones or dusty pastels. Add some chic sneaks or slides and a pair of sleek sunglasses in black or tortoise-shell, and you're ready to run from the playground to that potluck dinner with ease.

For slightly dressier days, add a short tan suede jacket that hits at your hip, and accent with a colorful scarf tied around your neck.

Finally, all good moms know that you can't get anywhere in life without a duffel bag the size of a minivan to tote around all the "necessities:" pacifiers, baby bottles, books, toys, snacks, diapers, cell phone, etc. A suede or leather tote bag is a smart investment, since it will carry all those mom and kid essentials and endure endless tossings into the car. If your budget doesn't allow for that, a black nylon tote will work just as well.

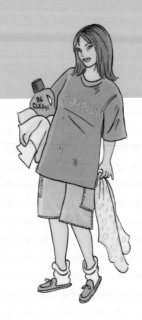

In just fifteen minutes, you've gone from World's Greatest Mom to World's Foxiest Mom!

~Foxy Hair~

Life is complicated enough for moms, so keep hair easy. Invest in a cut that takes minimal upkeep. To prevent split ends, ask your stylist for a look that won't require daily blow-drying. "Wash 'n go" is the salvation of many a busy mom. If you can, budget a few hours every six weeks or so for a little "you" time, when you can have your hair cut and colored, and maybe even splurge on a manicure or facial. Foxy moms deserve a treat every once in a while!

~Foxy Face and Bod~

Makeup needs to be not only easy but hearty enough to last through a day of chasing toddlers—or teenagers, as the case may be. Top off the Foxy Five with a bit of extra cover-up under the eyes where those hours of lost sleep are starting to show up. On days when your skin needs a pick-me-up, dot translucent shimmer stick on your forehead and cheekbones. Keep your lips looking soft and glossy with a tube of tinted lip balm.

Since motherhood comes with lots of inevitable diaper changing, kid bathing, toy toting, dish washing, and other things that can be hard on your hands, make sure you always carry along a tube of hand cream to moisturize. Look for something rich with coconut oil; it smells yummy, too. Try to find one that's anti-bacterial.

Foxy Finishing Touches

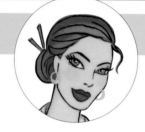

~Customizing It~

Now that you have the Foxy Formula down, turn things up by making it your own. You can maximize the number of looks by getting creative with accessories. Whip up your own personal brand of foxiness. The last thing you want is to look like you didn't put any imagination into getting ready, so put your stamp on it, Foxy!

Sooner or later, something will speak to you and work its way into your foxy style, whether it's a scent or a scarf. Here are a few ways foxettes add their own signature spin:

- **Themes:** daisies, bees, polka dots, Asian, Moroccan, African
- **Color:** purple, pink, green, black, or whatever hue suits you
- **Scent:** store bought or custom made for you and you only
- **Lipstick**: paint up your own personal palette of custom foxy shades
- **Scarves:** silk or wool, worn around your head, neck, or waist
- **Belts:** thin or thick, equestrian to ethnic
- **Jewelry:** hippie chokers, earrings, pins, brooches, bangles

- **Vintage:** purses, jewelry, jackets, scarves
- **Hats:** baseball, beret, straw, cowboy
- **Bags:** fringed, beaded, embellished, girly
- **Shoes:** boots, sneakers, sandals, stilettos, pumps, and on and on
- **Jackets:** jean, bomber, leather, collarless, safari
- **Coats:** trench, belted, embroidered
- **Sunglasses:** oversized, wrap, cat-eye, colorful
- **Watches:** men's style, oversized, athletic, diamond, vintage

All foxettes have that favorite item of clothing, whether it's a suede jacket or alligator skin pumps, that they will love—and wear—to death. Whatever you fancy, Foxy, own it and strut your stuff!

~All Day Foxiness~

It's one thing to put yourself together in the morning and look foxy as you leave the house, but cut to later that day, and your foxiness may be starting to fade.

We foxettes are always on the go, so we have to find ways to keep ourselves foxy from morning 'til night. We've come up with five "on the go" kits we never want to be caught without:

~ **The Foxy Handbag Kit.** There are so many times that we live out of our bags, so make sure your daily tote is filled with a few essentials: mini hand-sanitizing gel, all-in-one makeup stick, neutral lip gloss, tissues, blotting paper, mints.

~ **The Foxy Road Kit.** For many of us, our cars are like our second homes, so stock your sedan or SUV with staples: sunscreen, brush, tissues, lip balm, hand cream, baby wipes, toothpicks, mints, travel umbrella.

~ **The Foxy Office Kit.** Since you may spend eight hours or more a day at the office, keep a stash of goodies on hand to help you stay glammed up all day: dental floss, hand-sanitizing gel, toothbrush and toothpaste, pain reliever, cover-up, blush, colored lip gloss, perfume.

~ **The Foxy Flight Kit.** Fly high with a foxy "first aid" kit: lip gloss, facial mist, face and body moisturizer, mints, toothbrush, travel-size toothpaste, bottled water, cashmere or cotton socks, baby wipes, earplugs, moisturizing eye drops, inflatable pillow.

~ **The Foxy Gym Kit.** Add weight to your workout with a foxy fit kit: cover-up, all-in-one color stick, lip gloss, deodorant, hair elastics, headbands or clips, fresh fitted T-shirt.

Well, now you've got everything you need to take the world by storm, Foxy. It doesn't matter whether you're walking the dog or being wooed by Mr. Right, dredging through a kickboxing class or digging into a bowl of sorbet at home, lounging poolside or partying with friends—you can be foxy anytime, anywhere in just fifteen minutes flat!

stila

Get Foxy with stila!

stila has whipped up a gorgeous, easy to use Frumpy to Foxy Collection available exclusively at www.stilacosmetics.com. Go online and discover stila's Foxy Five beauty essentials, sure to make you Foxy...fast!

Foxy Eyes:
> Shadow Pots
> Major Lash Mascara
> Convertible Lash Line

Foxy Cheeks:
> Convertible Color for cheeks and lips
> Rouge Pots

Foxy Lips:
> Lip Glaze
> Twinsets

Foxy Face:
> Sheer Color Tinted Moisturizer with SPF 15
> Pivotal Skin
> Loose Powder

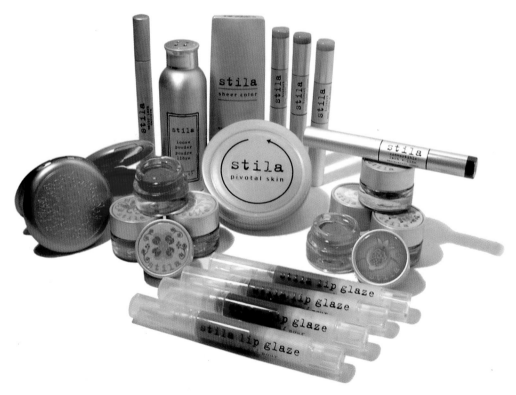